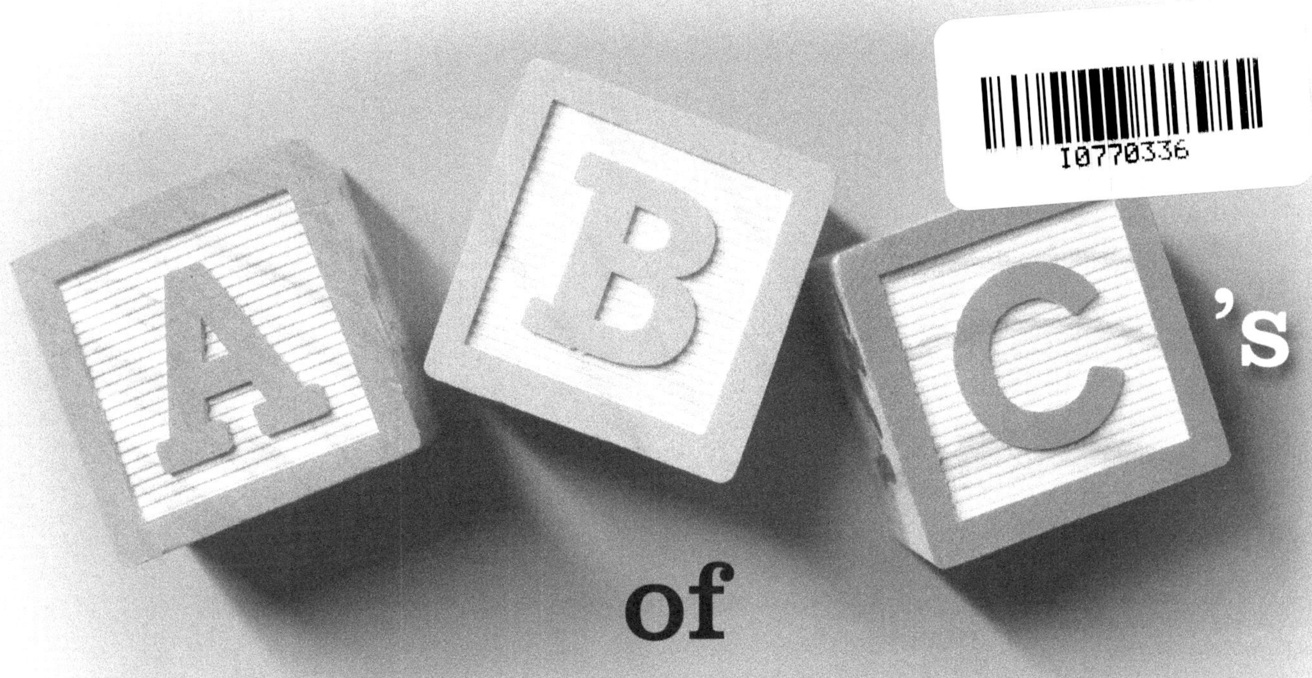

of

HEAD INJURY

EANE HUFF, M.S.

Table of Contents

SAGE Advice

Before we begin, let me say a bit about **SAGE** [**S**afety **A**llows **G**rieving and **E**mpowerment] advice. This acronym is found within all four books because of its significance. It will be useful in specific ways along each step. At this first stage, it narrows in on safety. Trauma changes the brain. But by following the **SAGE** steps, you can often correct the brain's changes.

Wise advice is an essential part of the healing process. Hopper [1], quotes Herman in Herman's Stages of Recovery. According to Hopper[2], trauma starts with **SAGE** advice:

Safety—

Dependability, predictability, and strength start a trauma recovery. According to Hopper[3], key aspects of safety in recovery include, "tapping into one's inner strengths…any other potentially available resources for healing…personal safety, genuine self-care, and healthy emotion regulation capacities" (pp1-2). According to Hopper[4], "…safety, stability and self-regulation…" (p. 3) are the skills of this first level. Therefore, in the first manual, *Heads Up*, we help acquaint the brain with an approved model for brain injury recovery success.

Allowing—

Peer relationships are involved in breakthroughs in recovery. Relationships allow individuals to overcome their trauma. Talking and relating to others allows the brain to heal. *ABCs of Recovery*, this second book in this quadrilogy, focuses on maximizing the benefit of relationships in recovery.

Grieving—

According to Hopper[5], "methods involve re-experiencing the memories within a safe and healing therapy setting. This can be very effective at ending the influence of such memories

---

1   Herman's Stages of Recovery: A three stage model of recovery from traumatic experiences, including sexual abuse and assault. Retrieved from: https://1in6.org/men/get-information/online-readings/recovery-and-therapy/stages-of-recovery/ Retrieved on 11-12-2016.

2   Herman's Stages of Recovery: A three stage model of recovery from traumatic experiences, including sexual abuse and assault. Retrieved from: https://1in6.org/men/get-information/online-readings/recovery-and-therapy/stages-of-recovery/ Retrieved on 11-12-2016.

3   Herman's Stages of Recovery: A three stage model of recovery from traumatic experiences, including sexual abuse and assault. Retrieved from: https://1in6.org/men/get-information/online-readings/recovery-and-therapy/stages-of-recovery/ Retrieved on 11-12-2016.

4   Herman's Stages of Recovery: A three stage model of recovery from traumatic experiences, including sexual abuse and assault. Retrieved from: https://1in6.org/men/get-information/online-readings/recovery-and-therapy/stages-of-recovery/ Retrieved on 11-12-2016.

5   Herman's Stages of Recovery: A three stage model of recovery from traumatic experiences, including sexual abuse and assault. Retrieved from: https://1in6.org/men/get-information/online-readings/recovery-and-therapy/stages-of-recovery/ Retrieved on 11-12-2016.

in one's life" (p. 3). Grieving is an important part of the recovery process, and strong leadership can further assist you in the journey. The third book in this series, *Discovering Yourself: Flight Plans*, incorporates identifying missing parts of self to draw upon leadership empowerment to thrive in recovery.

Empowerment—

To help others, according to Hopper[6], "…this stage of recovery focuses on *reconnecting* with people, meaningful activities, and other aspects of life" (p. 4). Empowerment helps us continue our healing past trauma by following our success. By completing *Creative Healing*, an additional book in this series, we start to allow ourselves to see what opens to us after the trauma.

These steps restore healing and internal balance to a survivor of head injury. They also allow grieving and acceptance of personal losses while adding an empowering part of living. These changes enhance life and add to an essential part of being Human. Relying on **SAGE** advice to heal from trauma deals with Safety, which can be expressed with these 5 questions:

1. How are you tapping into your inner strengths?
2. What level of safety are you providing that is adjusted to how you need to feel to recover?
3. What genuine types of self-care are you developing to assist your recovery?
4. How are you regulating your recovery achievement with stability and accurate expectations?
5. What other changes are you making for a successful recovery from trauma?

One last essential reminder as you apply the information in this quadrilogy: Partnering with your doctors and professional team in your recovery from trauma is encouraged and responsible. Do not apply any recovery practices without confirming they will be safe for you personally.

---

6 Herman's Stages of Recovery: A three stage model of recovery from traumatic experiences, including sexual abuse and assault. Retrieved from: https://1in6.org/men/get-information/online-readings/recovery-and-therapy/stages-of-recovery/ Retrieved on 11-12-2016.

Maps to Recovery and Healing

Relationships guide the brain toward healing. The brain is dependent on its owner to guide it toward the relationship opportunities it yearns for. The sequence of books of *HEADS UP, ABCs of Head Injury, Discovering Yourself: FLIGHT PLANS,* and *Creative Healing* will help a successful recovery emerge. While you may not understand the eagerness you feel toward peer relationships right now, the way you relate with peers demonstrates how the brain is trying to heal and rehabilitate itself from trauma as you familiarize yourself with the symptoms of your specific head injury. Working with the aspects of relationships to heal trauma starts a foundation of recovery that will be beneficial to work from.

While you may feel saddened by an inability to connect with your peers—brought by the complications of head injury—the choice to learn from the experiences and from your feelings will enable you to have a better idea of what challenges you. The feelings you get are accurate indicators that you have experienced a head injury and are struggling with the friendship and social areas of brain injury. How you relate and value your relationships with your peers can reveal how much success or failure you are having when dealing with the matter of the social dimension of relating. Healing trauma and finding relationship proficiency will best be achieved when you find your peer group. If you feel stunted, withdrawn, or unable to express yourself, it may not be your peer group!

I have found my peer group in a brain injury support group and heal with it at least once a week. I realize how different all our situations are, but I also realize how I'm healing by attending the meetings. Finding that peer group is a spectacular celebration! You will be participating in therapy and rehabilitation by engaging in peer relationships and learning, listening, and supporting others! I feel the healing as I participate. I connect with the healing of participating in peer relationships. It is where you find your peer group that will allow and encourage you to heal your trauma and succeed with healing. Find the way past trauma. The peer group is an essential part of healing and benefits those who search for it.

The connections that are made between individuals rely on confident communication skills, according to Poole Heller.[7] "The ability to relate with a wide variety of individuals comfortably and with confidence can mean a more connected, tolerant, and harmonious community…" (p. 2). This harmony brings better, healing health to the brain. Attachments are the healing stuff for brain trauma.

---

7   Poole Heller (n.d.). How Secure Attachment Fosters a Healthy Community. Retrieved on: 5-21-2018. Retrieved from: https://dianepooleheller.com/secure-attachment-fosters-healthy-community/.

The communication skills that will act as a bridge to getting you to the healing with your peers is learning how to **STOP** and communicate:

Small talk—begin with questions or tell another person you appreciate them

Talk about facts, make a comment about the situation

Opinions—move into voicing your opinions

Personal statement—finally, a statement that sums up the conversation or opens the possibility of establishing another one sometime later

This progression of communication allows a confident approach toward establishing communications that will be healing to the trauma sustained from the head injury. By continuing to **STOP** and communicate, you will become more confident in your personal style and help to heal yourself! Encouraging confident communications with your peers, you discover healing and encourage harmony within yourself.

Finding Harmony with Relationships and Healing Trauma

Experiencing a brain injury may have caused considerable damage and created an uphill battle for people recovering from this type of trauma. One of the most important building blocks in recovery, and one that is often overlooked or omitted completely, is the process of socialization during recovery from trauma. Neglecting relationships severely limits any recovery because of how essential attachments are to growth.

Consider this: those doing the best in dealing with trauma may not be the ones who have received the best therapies or worked the hardest at their recovery exercises. Instead, those excelling at their recovery may be the individuals with the most secure attachments. Secure attachments start the brain's process of working with trauma. According to Brickel and Associates,[8] "Deep relationships are essential…for trauma survivors" (p. 2). Relationships (also called attachments) are the foundation of healing trauma.

The ABCs of Head Injury are essential relationship skills that will change your trauma and change your life. One relationship skill for every letter of the alphabet.

---

8   Brickel and Associates (n.d.). Retrieved on 4-25-2018. Retrieved from: https://brickelandassociates.com/healing-relationships-after-trauma/.

ATTACHMENT TYPES

According to Hussey,[9] "The three main attachment types most of us adopt are secure, anxious, and avoidant" (p. 2). Each attachment style will influence how we deal with trauma and the associations made with others which may bring comfort. Hussey[10] claims that "those with a secure style feel equally okay with displaying interest and affection, and being alone and independent. They can cope with rejection and are less prone to obsessing over their relationships" (p. 2).

The second type of attachment style is anxious.[11] "Those with an anxious attachment style… need plenty of reassurance from their partners. They have difficulty in being single compared with the other two styles" (p. 2).

The third attachment style is avoidant. A challenging mix of feelings are represented in this relationship style.[12] Avoidant types are "independent, self-referencing, and usually uncomfortable with intimacy. They may avoid commitment and/or construct their lifestyle in such a way to avoid too much contact with their partners" (p. 3).

A fourth, additional type of attachment[13] is the "anxious-avoidant attachment style…relatively rare…. It is a style best characterized by conflicting desires: to be close but also push people away. [There is] evidence of low psychological health in other areas of their life; for example, there may be issues with substance abuse and depression" (p. 3).

Out of these four attachment styles, which do you think could handle the needs of trauma the best? More importantly, are you that attachment style or do you know which attachment style you are? Are you finding any idiosyncrasies that are inhibiting your recovery from trauma? How can you try to compensate for those? If the healing journey with trauma is from relationships, which are essential to trauma survivors, how can you work with your attachment style to find success?

ACTION SIGNALS

Taking action is how to connect with trauma and recovery. Trauma causes such a paralysis to the human mind, and action signals from negative emotions may be the keys that hold the hidden messages that the mind may not be ready to register. According to JD,[14] "Every emotion has a message for you. Appreciate the message. Negative emotions are a signal that change is needed" (p. 1).

---

9   Hussey (2018). 14 Things You Need to Know about Adult Attachment Theory. Retrieved on: 4-25-2018. Retrieved from: http://www.artofwellbeing.com/2016/09/02/attachmenttheory/.

10   Hussey (2018). 14 Things You Need to Know about Adult Attachment Theory. Retrieved on: 4-25-2018. Retrieved from: http://www.artofwellbeing.com/2016/09/02/attachmenttheory/.

11   Hussey (2018). 14 Things You Need to Know about Adult Attachment Theory. Retrieved on: 4-25-2018. Retrieved from: http://www.artofwellbeing.com/2016/09/02/attachmenttheory/.

12   Hussey (2018). 14 Things You Need to Know about Adult Attachment Theory. Retrieved on: 4-25-2018. Retrieved from: http://www.artofwellbeing.com/2016/09/02/attachmenttheory/.

13   Hussey (2018). 14 Things You Need to Know about Adult Attachment Theory. Retrieved on: 4-25-2018. Retrieved from: http://www.artofwellbeing.com/2016/09/02/attachmenttheory/.

14   JD (n.d.). Use Negative Emotions as a Call to Action. Retrieved on: 4-28-2018. Retrieved from: http://sourcesofinsight.com/action-signals-use-negative-emotions-as-a-call-to-action/.

Each emotion can carry a meaning. According to JD,[15] "At any moment when you feel any negative emotion, the first step is to identify the Action Signal…. The next step, after you identify the Action Signal, is to take action by either changing your perception or changing your procedure" (p. 1).

The action signals express a need that the individual is feeling. They express the emotions that inspire a need for something. What have your emotions told you that you have **HAD LONGING** for?

Hurt[16]—"Hurt reflects a sense of loss…you have a need that is not being met" (p. 2-4).

Anger[17]—Anger shows a person is "mildly irritated…" (p. 2).

Disappointment[18]—Disappointment reflects "sad, defeated" feelings.

Loneliness[19]—Loneliness reflects a feeling of being "apart or separate from" (p. 2).

Overwhelmed[20]—Being overwhelmed reflects being "hopeless or depressed" (p. 2).

Needs comfort[21]—Being uncomfortable reflects a person who is "impatient, uneasy, distressed, mildly embarrassed" (p. 2).

Guilt[22]—Feeling guilty reflects "emotions or regret" (p. 2).

Inadequacy[23]—Inadequacy reflects "[feeling less] than or unworthy" (p. 2).

Needs safety[24]—Action signals that reflect the need of safety reflect emotions like "impatient, uneasy, distressed, mildly embarrassed" (p. 2).

Great frustration[25]—Action signals indicating frustration reflect feeling "held back or hindered in the pursuit of something" (p. 2).

---

15 JD (n.d.). Use Negative Emotions as a Call to Action. Retrieved on: 4-28-2018. Retrieved from: http://sourcesofinsight.com/action-signals-use-negative-emotions-as-a-call-to-action/.
16 JD (n.d.). Use Negative Emotions as a Call to Action. Retrieved on: 4-28-2018. Retrieved from: http://sourcesofinsight.com/action-signals-use-negative-emotions-as-a-call-to-action/.
17 JD (n.d.). Use Negative Emotions as a Call to Action. Retrieved on: 4-28-2018. Retrieved from: http://sourcesofinsight.com/action-signals-use-negative-emotions-as-a-call-to-action/.
18 JD (n.d.). Use Negative Emotions as a Call to Action. Retrieved on: 4-28-2018. Retrieved from: http://sourcesofinsight.com/action-signals-use-negative-emotions-as-a-call-to-action/.
19 JD (n.d.). Use Negative Emotions as a Call to Action. Retrieved on: 4-28-2018. Retrieved from: http://sourcesofinsight.com/action-signals-use-negative-emotions-as-a-call-to-action/.
20 JD (n.d.). Use Negative Emotions as a Call to Action. Retrieved on: 4-28-2018. Retrieved from: http://sourcesofinsight.com/action-signals-use-negative-emotions-as-a-call-to-action/.
21 JD (n.d.). Use Negative Emotions as a Call to Action. Retrieved on: 4-28-2018. Retrieved from: http://sourcesofinsight.com/action-signals-use-negative-emotions-as-a-call-to-action/.
22 JD (n.d.). Use Negative Emotions as a Call to Action. Retrieved on: 4-28-2018. Retrieved from: http://sourcesofinsight.com/action-signals-use-negative-emotions-as-a-call-to-action/.
23 JD (n.d.). Use Negative Emotions as a Call to Action. Retrieved on: 4-28-2018. Retrieved from: http://sourcesofinsight.com/action-signals-use-negative-emotions-as-a-call-to-action/.
24 JD (n.d.). Use Negative Emotions as a Call to Action. Retrieved on: 4-28-2018. Retrieved from: http://sourcesofinsight.com/action-signals-use-negative-emotions-as-a-call-to-action/.
25 JD (n.d.). Use Negative Emotions as a Call to Action. Retrieved on: 4-28-2018. Retrieved from: http://sourcesofinsight.com/action-signals-use-negative-emotions-as-a-call-to-action/.

These action signals all carry a need with them. Each emotion we have is notifying us that the relationship with our needs is not satisfied. It is time to find what those emotions mean and satisfy them.

BELIEF

Belief is more than a concept in living: having a belief is fundamental. Beliefs are what you return to after your accomplishments are done, when the challenges are over, and when it is time to turn in for the night.

Because beliefs are so essential in a head injury recovery, it is important to find the beliefs that work for you. Which beliefs work best? That depends on what you want to achieve. If you need higher self-esteem, positive beliefs should be worked into your life. If you aim to be more active, emphasis on action may be essential. If people are wanted in your life, then the belief that associations are important should be increased.

Beliefs determine and direct behavior. You will find your beliefs transfer to the behavior you have. According to Taghavi,[26] "Your actions primarily carry out orders from your subconscious programming, and the way you invest in yourself, how deserving and entitled you believe yourself to be—creates indirect communication and other unconscious signals to the world around you and everyone you come into contact with in your day to day life" (p. 1).

The beliefs you operate with are very indicative of how you choose to operate. They indicate how much you will be motivated to expend effort toward achieving a goal. Your beliefs will make you extend extra effort to represent those beliefs. While addressing looking for a relationship after a head injury, how you believe you deserve your relationship is an important factor. According to Taghavi,[27] "Believing you deserve is half the battle to getting what you want, so act the part, believe you deserve and invest in yourself" (p. 3).

---

26 Taghavi (n.d.) You Get In Life What You Believe You Deserve—Here's How To Upgrade That Belief. Retrieved on 5-5-2018. Retrieved from https://medium.com/swlh/you-get-in-life-what-you-believe-you-deserve-heres-how-to-upgra...

27 Taghavi (n.d.) You Get In Life What You Believe You Deserve—Here's How To Upgrade That Belief. Retrieved on 5-5-2018. Retrieved from https://medium.com/swlh/you-get-in-life-what-you-believe-you-deserve-heres-how-to-upgra...

Peer Experience with Belief

The beliefs that I used to have compared to the beliefs I have now demonstrate a difference between how I view my attachments and also how much I extend myself to make a point of showing what I think makes a good relationship. Visiting the library today, I sat down at the computers. There was an empty seat beside me, which was quickly taken by a library patron. I welcomed her to the library and told her that I hoped she was having a good day. By welcoming her like that, I believe I opened the possibilities for her to ask me a question because she was relatively new at using computers. I gave her the answer, and her smile widened because she was relieved. When I welcomed her to the library, I extended what I believed should be put forth during a meeting. I wasn't trying to do what I thought the person might need. I extended what I believed a good relationship needed. I didn't try to change myself or my presentation; I just was an original representation of the person I believe I need to be. I achieved what I thought was representative of friendship behavior, and by investing in that friendship behavior, I invested in what I thought would be representative of who I am. I behaved like my beliefs showed me I should treat relationships, and I opened a door of friendship with a person who I was friendly with.

Bowen Family Systems Theory

Bowen family systems theory is a theory about communication and relationships. Relationships are essential to the recovery process, so it is helpful to have a healthy sense about relationship difficulties and possible detractions.

Relationships, according to Bowen family systems, can be expressed in triangles. According to Brown,[28] "Triangling is said to occur when…anxiety in a dyad is relieved by…a third party…who either takes sides or provides a detour for the anxiety" (p. 3).

This anxiety felt from your partner in communication may not be something you can control. All you can do is understand the situation that is often experienced by people who are talking, and recognize how it may not be the best communication situation. This is where you can find a lot of reliance on your beliefs, because it can be as important to display communication that is consistent with your belief of how you should treat people.

---

28 Brown (n.d.). Retrieved on 5-5-2018. Retrieved from: http://www.thefsi.com.au/wp-content/uuploads/2014/01/Bowen-family-Systems-Theory-and-Practice_Illustrations-and -Critique.pdf. Retrieved on 5-5-2018.

> **Peer experience with Bowen family systems theory**
>
> **Triangling can occur when communicating with others who don't quite seem to be getting the message—when other's apprehensions or anxiety seem to be distorting the message or interfering with what people are understanding from your communicating with them. By approaching communication nervously, your communication partners will not understand or acknowledge your message. Triangling complicates the message that you are giving and makes communication for people who have experienced a head injury discouraging. But by communicating as best you can, you will find a way through triangling and find a way to better relationships.**

COGNITIVE RESTRUCTURING

Surviving a head injury is just part of the challenge; changing to meet the needs of your recovery is the next step to ensure a high quality of life. The experience of a head injury can be traumatic in many ways. It can leave disabilities; it can cause a change in your life, and those changes may be negatively interpreted. This is where cognitive restructuring holds benefits to recovery and rehabilitation; it changes your day to success! Cognitive restructuring, according to Mind Tools,[29] "…helps you to change negative or distorted thinking that often lies behind…moods. As such, it helps you approach situations in a more positive frame of mind" (p. 2). Dealing with negative subjects with a positive frame of mind allows success to be taken from the situations. Instead of looking at a situation in negative terms, you allow yourself to see and build on the positives that happen in every recovery. The following are key points to cognitive restructuring, according to Mind Tools[30]:

Calm yourself.

Write down the situation that triggered the negative thoughts.

Identify the moods that you felt in the situation.

Write down the automatic thoughts you experienced when you felt the mood. The most significant of these are your "hot thoughts."

Identify the evidence that supports these hot thoughts.

Identify the evidence that contradicts the hot thoughts.

Now, identify fair, balanced thoughts about the situation.

Finally, observe your mood now, and decide on your next steps.

---

29   Mind Tools (n.d.) Cognitive Restructuring: Reducing Stress by Changing Your Thinking. Retrieved on 5-5-2018. Retrieved from: https://www.mindtools.com/pages/article/new/TCS_81.htm.

30   Mind Tools (n.d.) Cognitive Restructuring: Reducing Stress by Changing Your Thinking. Retrieved on 5-5-2018. Retrieved from: https://www.mindtools.com/pages/article/new/TCS_81.htm.

Go through this process when you experience a negative mood, or when you feel fear, apprehension, or anxiety about a person or event (p. 6).

Peer Experience: Cognitive Restructuring

Relationship issues are some of the toughest issues to deal with. Distorted expectations and reactions concerning a highly valuable relationship mean that emotions can be highly reactive when trying to participate and succeed in them. But, by recognizing your emotions and being able to write about them, you make yourself a participant in learning about relationships, able to get past the negativity that can result from difficult experiences and learning from a head injury.

Cognitive restructuring works for things beyond relationships. Using cognitive restructuring to find the positives of recovery despite a few negatives allows a truly balanced approach to rehabilitation. By allowing yourself to get past the difficult emotions and not get stuck in a mood, you achieve beyond what could be limiting and restrictive to recovery potential. By choosing to use cognitive restructuring in your recovery, you give yourself options to recognize the positives and negatives of the recovery process. Then you enable yourself to get past it.

COMORBIDITY

Comorbidity is a challenge to relationships because it involves more maintenance than what only dealing with one disability involves. According to Dictionary.com,[31] "comorbid means pertaining to two diseases which occur together, such as ADHD and depression" (p. 2).

Head injuries are likely to cause comorbid conditions. Depression from head injury may cause reliance on addictive substances, resulting in a comorbid condition.

Recovery gets complicated. The relationship emphasis when dealing with trauma is reprioritized to finding ways to work with relationships, which is already a problem area for many survivors. Your priorities suffer, and you do not commit enough to your relationship paradigm to heal the trauma. Your brain does not take full advantage of healing trauma because you are unable to give attention to the relationship.

---

31   Dictionary.com (n.d.) Comorbid, Retrieved on 5-7-2018. Retrieved from: http://www.dictionary.com/.

> **Peer Experience: Comorbidity**
>
> **The challenge of realizing comorbidity and being able to prioritize the needs of disabilities compares with how you attend to your relationships. Depression will be a common disability to deal with, yet trying to establish a relationship while depressed is not something that will bring an optimal outcome.**
>
> **The priorities that I extend toward dealing with my disabilities have changed according to my acceptance of who I am. A visual disability and the paralyzed half of my body don't allow me to manage my appearance. If I miss my collar being turned idiosyncratically, that's too bad, but it's who I really am. The relationships that stick with me despite what may turn out as odd are the relationships that I can really count on.**
>
> **Comorbidity is a real impediment to recovery and rehabilitation for people who struggle with multiple disabilities. It steals focus and can make relationships harder than they once were. Acceptance of self is usually one of the hardest and longest processes of head injury recovery, but it is especially helpful for dealing with comorbid conditions. Your relationship skills will benefit because you will be able to concentrate on revealing who you truly are.**

CONTROLLED DEFIANCE

Controlled defiance is an exceptional recovery tool. It operates from a philosophy of, according to Pottenger,[32] controlled defiance, which "includes the possibility of change: resisting environment and instinct; rising above any conditions fate may deal to us…we can choose…. what we are, what we become. Healthy people believe that they can change" (p. 1). Controlled defiance relies on that belief that change can happen, and takes power from the decision to change. Deciding to be different than who you were, or deciding to stay the same despite the circumstances, really does bring health and a sense of control to the circumstances.

---

32 Pottenger (nd). Viktor Frankl and the Human Search for Meaning. Retrieved on: 5-12-2018. Retrieved from: http://www. Ccrsdodona.org/m_dilemma/1982/pis/frankl.html

Peer Experience Controlled Defiance:

Controlled defiance is something that can make your recovery yours. It gives you back a feeling of self-direction, a feeling that you own your success. Recovery becomes personal and that actually does encourage a personal reinvestment of self. By choosing what to do or who to be, you become healthy and invested into recovery.

The choice to be how you feel or who you are is such a strong choice in recovery. It is also a necessary choice, because the choice to return to the power of who you actually are is so important. Acceptance of who you are becomes paramount. As you use more of yourself to achieve the best recovery, you display more of yourself! And feel ownership of your recovery!

DISCOVERY

Discovery is a skill that involves being the **REF** of your game of success. It involves **R**esponsibility, **E**xpectations, and **F**eedback. The blend of these three concepts makes Discovery an essential recovery tool.

Responsibility, according to the OASIS movement:[33] "…being responsible means doing what needs to be done, when it needs to be done. It means setting priorities and taking action on them" (p. 1). Discovery of recovery opportunities and priorities means that recovery will be taken on as soon as it is available to engage in, and it will take a priority in rehabilitation to get better. Becoming accustomed to the opportunities that become available to recovering individuals is so important to grasp and take advantage of. Being in the flow of recovery does help immensely to become aware of timing and opportunity.

Expectations influence the amount of reward that is allowed to be felt. Too high of expectations, and you risk not experiencing a feeling of reward, while with too low of expectations, you risk not challenging yourself enough. But if you balance your expectations, you can assure yourself rewarding and positive experiences. According to Tugend,[34] "…there is a physiological reason we are disappointed when life does not meet our expectations. The neurotransmitter dopamine is released in our brain—and makes us feel good—when something positive happens" (p. 2). That dopamine is essential to feeling rewarded and fulfilled. The expectations that we each have are so essential to determining the level of reward we each obtain. It is important to monitor our expectations so that we can feel rewarded. Nothing should be too easy or too hard, but there

---

33 OASIS movement (n.d.). The Benefits of Being Responsible. Retrieved on: 5-12-2018. Retrieved from: http://www.Oasismovement.org/the-benefits-of-being-responsible/.

34 Tugend (2012). What Did You Expect? It Makes A Difference. Retrieved on 5-12-2018. Retrieved from:www.nytimes.com/2012/01/14/your-money/the-importance-of-setting-expectations-whethe…

should be an element of challenge that will push your potential to rise to the top.

Feedback is used to determine both our own responsibility and expectations. According to How to Use Feedback to Recover from Stroke Faster,[35] "…Feedback…is really important for your recovery" (p. 1). Feedback will allow you to adjust your responsibility and expectations to discover the best of yourself. Feedback will allow you to adjust your approach, adjust your attitude, and be present with any of the demands of a successful recovery. Being the **REF** of your game of success does allow Discovery of how easy you can make the recovery process on yourself. Take responsibility to realize your personal time to recover, to realize the proper amount of expectations, and finally, to understand the results that a successful recovery needs. By doing all three steps, you have just allowed discovery of a better recovery.

Peer Experience: Discovery

Discovery contains the aspects of a successful recovery. Being the REF of your own game of success involves using the responsibility to engage in recovery, the use of expectations to fully experience reward and fulfillment that includes achieving what we expect of ourselves, and using feedback to successfully understand where our recovery's progress is.

This three-part formula of allowing recovery to succeed is integral to peer concepts. Responsibility will allow you to engage in parts of your recovery that are important to you, expectations will allow you to feel fulfilled and rewarded, which can impact your attitude toward others, and the feedback you receive from your recovery will allow you to find what peer group you want to belong to according to your abilities and success.

Discovery allows the detection of who you are in your recovery. It will give you focus about who you want to be and will show you the responsibility which can show you the best of your recovery. Discovery isn't just a concept that reveals your potential self by unearthing recovery tools; discovery is what can allow you to become the best you can be and become a leader among your peers.

*E*MOTIONAL *I*NTELLIGENCE

Emotional intelligence is an important concept in peer experiences. According to Healthy Sense of Self,[36] "Emotional intelligence has to do with your self-awareness and ability to manage your emotions while helping others manage theirs" (p. 2).

This peer awareness and response can be difficult for those dealing with limited sensory intake

---

35 How to Use Feedback to Recover from Stroke Faster. (2017). Retrieved on 5-12-2018. Retrieved from: https://www.flintrehab.com/2017/feedback-for-stroke-recovery/.

36 Healthy Sense of Self (2018).What Is Emotional Intelligence and Why Does It Matter? Retrieved on 5-14-2018. Retrieved from: https://healthysenseofself.com/22018/04/emotional-intelligence/?gclid=EAIaIQobChMItljIt.

or different abilities. Emotional Intelligence has four parts[37]: "1. Have a keen awareness of the way you feel. 2. The ability to manage your emotions. 3. Be aware of other people's emotions. 4. The ability to manage and handle other's emotions" (p. 2-6).

Emotional intelligence is highly reliant upon the ability to be aware of emotions and demonstrate competence. It means that people who are emotionally intelligent give permission for others to be upset, to hurt, and they also allow them to return to a preferred state. The key emphasis is the reliance on understanding and handling your feelings and being able to manage and handle other's emotions. This can be very important when people are dealing with trauma.

An important ability is the ability to observe.[38] "…You can always improve and become more aware of the emotions you're experiencing, why they're coming up, and how you're showing up to the world. The important thing here is to be an impartial observer. You don't need to judge your feelings, just watch them arise" (p. 3).

Peer Experience with Emotional Intelligence

Emotional Intelligence is the key to fulfilling peer relationships and understanding what is needed in peer relationships. It allows watching traumatic emotions arise and realizing that they won't be of help, so you try your best to make it through them. Being emotionally intelligent is allowing the feelings you have exist within you, but not being affected by the emotions. It means being comfortable with the situation that peer relationships involve and being fine with it.

Emotional intelligence depends on having the confidence which will allow engagement with a conversation's demands and needs. By providing what you can, you already know what you feel you're good at and have a realization of how you can control your emotions. You find that while monitoring your emotions, you are also able to monitor other people's emotions. Finally, you're able to handle those emotions that come from others during the conversation.

Relaxing into an emotionally intelligent persona brings relaxation and acceptance that you're going to do the best you can and be aware of the most you can. Emotional intelligence is a definite skill that can be relied on in peer experiences.

---

37   Healthy Sense of Self (2018).What Is Emotional Intelligence and Why Does It Matter? Retrieved on 5-14-2018. Retrieved from: https://healthysenseofself.com/22018/04/emotional-intelligence/?gclid=EAIalQobChMltljlt.
38   Healthy Sense of Self (2018).What Is Emotional Intelligence and Why Does It Matter? Retrieved on 5-14-2018. Retrieved from: https://healthysenseofself.com/22018/04/emotional-intelligence/?gclid=EAIalQobChMltljlt.

S*ELF-E*STEEM

Self-Esteem is the survival technique that changes recovery. According to Psychology Today,[39] "Possessing little self-regard can lead people to become depressed, to fall short of their potential, or to tolerate abusive situations and relationships. Too much self-love, on the other hand, results in an off-putting sense of entitlement and an inability to learn from failures" (p. 1).

This concept deals with peer relationships. It encourages interacting with situations and the people who you are dealing with. Many times, a recovery concept that is being struggled with will adversely affect how you view yourself and your opportunities. The peers you have a chance to connect with and give encouraging support to may seem distant and uncaring.

That is the time when you need to check your self-esteem. You may be operating with too little acknowledgment of what you have been through. Or you may be operating with too much emphasis on what you have been through. The importance of self-esteem is adapting to what the situation needs. A peer struggling with recovery may not be ready to hear how your recovery is going unexpectedly well, but that peer may be waiting to hear how you want to join them on their therapy exercises and routine. Self-esteem is all about being ready to interact and provide what the situation needs. It's feeling good enough about yourself that you are able to find what the situation needs.

The biggest benefit and challenge of working with good self-esteem is to personal functioning. Taking the head injury and accepting it reveals a phenomenal recovery potential.

Peer Experience with Self-Esteem

Personal situations will be the most influencing toward peer relationships. Bad days or hard experiences will lessen self-esteem's ability to provide what the situation needs. Peer awareness and acceptance of self can be influenced by situations related to disability and other effects of the head injury. A speed of processing that is slower than others around you may frustrate you. It may make you limit the amount of interacting you do with your peer group. Self-esteem that is interactive, however, will encourage you to find a group with acceptance of your abilities. Good self-esteem will encourage you to become comfortable with your speed of processing and find benefits in what you can do. Incorporating the head injury's symptoms and using them to reveal your individual style is finding the optimal route to self-esteem.

---

39 https://www.psychology today.com/us/basics/self-esteem.

FEELINGS

Our feelings are clues to how we need to adjust the recovery practices and support we need as we engage in peer relationships and support. The feelings give us clues to the message beneath it. According to Inner Truth Studios,[40] "If we keep feeling the same emotion strongly, presumably it's a message we should listen to..." (p. 2). Our feelings are messengers that can enlighten each of us[41] if we "dive into our feelings and consciously pay close attention to our felt experience without labeling or analyzing it" (p. 2).

By understanding that our feelings are actually messages, we can understand emotional clues by paying close attention to personal feelings. Inner Truth Studios[42] reports, "Paying close attention to our feelings, emotions became messengers that lead us to a greater understanding of who we are and what we want to achieve" (p. 2). Viewing your feelings as clues to your life will enable you to understand more potential than ever before.

Peer Experience: Feelings

Feelings in recovery often become reactive instead of revealing. In resisting the impulse to react against emotions, it is important to ask, "What is this emotion telling me?" Maybe it's anxiety or frustration. How you answer it will be your success. How will you choose to look at your feelings and let them add to your recovery? Your feelings are messages that you are finding within your operation and recovery. It's time to add that understanding to your recovery and find a way to better understand yourself and your situation.

FLEXIBILITY

The choice of flexibility is demanding not only in recovery, but also in communication—relating to your peers and interacting with them and their message or finding that communication needs to be restricted to your point of view so that you can be clear to your communication partners. The resources that you will be working with will enable your flexibility with communication, as well as the topics you communicate about and who you're communicating with. Memory skills and disabilities can limit the competence you feel and the ability you demonstrate.

How you decide to approach your communication will influence your approach and, likely, what you will make available to yourself. Do you feel comfortable with any personal skills that you

---

40   Inner Truth Studios (n.d). The Power of Emotional Connection. Retrieved on: 5-14-2018. Retrieved from: https//innertruth.org/pdcast/the-power-of-emtional-connection-raphael-cushnir/.

41   Inner Truth Studios (n.d). The Power of Emotional Connection. Retrieved on: 5-14-2018. Retrieved from: https//innertruth.org/pdcast/the-power-of-emtional-connection-raphael-cushnir/.

42   Inner Truth Studios (n.d). The Power of Emotional Connection. Retrieved on: 5-14-2018. Retrieved from: https//innertruth.org/pdcast/the-power-of-emtional-connection-raphael-cushnir/.

might incorporate into your conversation? By keeping this in mind, you will enable yourself to go to your skills in conversation. Flexibility—it can change your communication.

Peer Experience: Flexibility

The choice to find confidence in what you can do with your communication skills is greatly improved when finding flexibility. The choice of entering into a communication and being reliant upon your partner to choose what they want to talk about is usually instigated first by a choice of whether you want to disclose your story, whether you want to listen, or whether you want to learn. Those three choices can influence your questions and your attention. Flexibility is truly the addition to the conversation you will value and need.

GIVING

Giving is a peer-influenced behavior that has many benefits. It activates brain mechanisms and can result in, according to Bea,[43] "health benefits associated with giving: lower blood pressure, increased self-esteem, less depression, lower stress levels, longer life, [and] greater happiness" (p. 2).

Giving influences the brain. According to Bea,[44] "Giving can create a 'warm glow,' activating regions in the brain associated with pleasure, connection with other people and trust…during gift-giving behaviors, humans secrete 'feel good' chemicals in our brains, such as serotonin (a mood-mediating chemical), dopamine (a feel-good chemical), and oxytocin (a compassion and bonding chemical)" (p. 3-4).

Giving is relationship behavior that rewards the person receiving as well as the individual giving. According to Bea,[45] "Giving stimulates the mesolimbic pathway, which is the reward center in the brain—releasing endorphins and creating what is known as the 'helper's high.'" Giving is the gift that gives back.

---

43 Bea (n.d.). Wanna Give? This Is Your Brain on a Helper's High. Retrieved on 5-14-2018. Retrieved from: https://health. Clevelandclinic.org/why-giving-is-good-for-your-health/.

44 Bea (n.d.) Wanna Give? This Is Your Brain on a Helper's High. Retrieved on 5-14-2018. Retrieved from: https://health. Clevelandclinic.org/why-giving-is-good-for-your-health/.

45 Bea (n.d.). Wanna Give? This Is Your Brain on a Helper's High. Retrieved on 5-14-2018. Retrieved from: https://health. Clevelandclinic.org/why-giving-is-good-for-your-health/.

Peer Experience: Giving

Giving is one of the most misunderstood sources of peer-oriented relationships. The practice of giving is a positive health benefit, and the changes and influences it brings can give so much influence to communication health. While the benefits of giving can be many, the requirements of giving have many considerations.

Giving interest and giving time is so much more important than what many people think of giving: advice. Offering interest and support is a completely different perspective than "giving advice." While giving someone advice may influence a defensive response from the person you're giving it to, giving your time or giving your support transmits a different message. Giving time or support is usually signaled by the question "How can I help?" It is joining another's interest, and giving of your time and support. When realizing that this is actually "giving," you also enable the reward mechanisms which enable the same type of health benefits that giving activates! Giving: it's a way to receive as well as contribute! Find the health benefits of joining others with a giving attitude.

GRATITUDE

Gratitude has many benefits that can impact recovery and relationships. The more you engage in being grateful, the more the practice will change your life. According to Morin,[46] "Whether you choose to write a few sentences in a gratitude journal, or simply take a moment to silently acknowledge all you have, giving thanks can transform your life... Gratitude opens the door to more relationships" (p. 1). By being grateful, you change your personal actions, which culminate in showing appreciation. According to Morin, [47] "Showing appreciation can help you win new friends" (p. 1).

A large part of peer relationships during head injury revolves around the relationship health of the person with a head injury. Being mentally healthy and free from negative emotions that encourage competition, comparisons, or resentment is necessary. According to Morin,[48] "Research confirms, gratitude reduces a multitude of toxic emotions, from envy and resentment to frustration and regret...grateful people are able to appreciate other people's accomplishments" (p. 1-2).

Gratitude also plays a major factor in determining how trauma affects an individual. "Research

---

46   Morin (n.d.) 7 Scientifically Proven Benefits of Gratitude. Retrieved on 5-14-2018. Retrieved from: https://www.psychologyto-day.com/us/blog/what-mentally-strong-people-dont-do/2201504/...

47   Morin (n.d.) 7 Scientifically Proven Benefits of Gratitude. Retrieved on 5-14-2018. Retrieved from: https://www.psychologyto-day.com/us/blog/what-mentally-strong-people-dont-do/2201504/...

48   Morin (n.d.) 7 Scientifically Proven Benefits of Gratitude. Retrieved on 5-14-2018. Retrieved from: https://www.psychologyto-day.com/us/blog/what-mentally-strong-people-dont-do/2201504/...

has shown gratitude not only reduces stress, but it may play a major role in overcoming trauma… gratitude plays a major role in resilience" (p. 2).[49]

Peer Experience: Gratitude

Gratitude has such relevance to peer relationships and helping overcome trauma. The practice of gratitude encourages relationships that will help trauma recovery, and gratitude encourages the resilience that can help to foundationally counteract trauma.

Gratitude is a skill that will influence trauma recovery by adding so many aspects influencing social support. The proactive aspects of choosing gratitude allow a person to: increase the number of relationships, experience mental health and the freedom of social comparison, and realize an amount of resilience from trauma. Being grateful is one of the first steps to finding success when dealing with trauma.

HAPPINESS

Happiness is the aspect of life experience that will encourage someone in recovery to find their sustaining emotion that reveals that they are finding something the brain needs. The happiness is not only a clue to what a person truly desires. It gives us direction of where we need to be. Happiness brings us to a closer approximation of what the recovery from trauma really needs. According to Psychology Today,[50] "…Happiness is not the result of bouncing from one joy to the next; achieving happiness typically involves times of considerable discomfort…genetic makeup, life circumstances, achievements, marital status, social relationships…all influence how happy you are. Or can be" (p. 1).

Letting the feelings of happiness guide your recovery can be a calming and reinforcing matter of adding direction to your recovery. If all people need happiness in their life, then it is time to become aware of how much happiness can add to your life. Happiness is the direction toward which you can point your recovery.

Finding long-term happiness is linking a concept or theme in your recovery to achieve what you need. While subsisting on happiness in a recovery can be a limiting factor that is reflective of the circumstances involved, finding activities and situations that bring happiness can be a direction to a person in recovery from a head injury and lead to discovery of a person's joy.

---

49   Morin (n.d.) 7 Scientifically Proven Benefits of Gratitude. Retrieved on 5-14-2018. Retrieved from: https://www.psychologyto-day.com/us/blog/what-mentally-strong-people-dont-do/2201504/…

50   Psychology Today (n.d.) Happiness. Retrieved on: 5-16-2018, Retrieved from: https://www.psychologytoday.com/us/basics/happiness.

Happiness

Happiness is the barometer that can lead an individual to a better recovery perspective. When you trust the brain's experience, happiness can actually lead to the discovery of rewarding activity. By following your own personal view of happiness, you enable yourself to live with a connection to who you can be.

Realizing your personal happiness can be the clue to a rewarding and more fulfilling recovery. When connecting events that bring happiness, understanding happiness is a clue to what you will be drawn to and will enable you to find motivation in your recovery and discover what living in your joy is like.

HEMISPHERE PROCESSING

The brain uses two hemispheres in the brain to accurately understand the environment and opportunities within the environment. According to Right Brain vs. Left Brain,[51] "…Structure and functions of the mind suggest that the two different sides of the brain control the different 'modes' of thinking. It also suggests that each of us prefers one mode over the other" (p. 1). The different modes of thinking and learning reside in the left brain and right brain:[52] The left brain handles "logical, sequential, rational, analytical, objective, looks at parts" (p. 2), while the right brain handles the "random, intuitive, holistic, synthesizing, subjective, looks at wholes" (p. 2).

These different processing styles reveal the effects of head injury and the brain's efforts to compensate for it. The brain will use its fastest hemisphere to process the environment, which means that the uninjured, fastest hemisphere will likely be the processing method that will be easiest for you.

When the brain is injured, it starts rewiring into the uninjured hemisphere. While the brain can easily subsist on only one hemisphere's processing and production, it does so much better experiencing and producing the vitality of life with two hemispheres. Because of the brain's amazing communication, it will notice if one hemisphere is operating slower than the other. It will start to reroute wiring and change predispositions. You will be more inclined to use the uninjured hemisphere in dealing with the environment. Yet the change will be so subtle, you probably won't even notice it.

Your processing style using the uninjured hemisphere will enable you to operate with your fastest, most responsive hemisphere. Yet even though it may be the fastest hemisphere, it may be the hemisphere that is not suited for the environment it is in. Your communication style will reflect this with how you relate to your peers. If your left hemisphere is injured, the right hemisphere will

---

51   Right Brain vs. Left Brain (n.d.). Retrieved on: 5-16-2018. Retrieved from: http://www.funderstanding.com/brain/right-brain-vs-left-brain/.
52   Right Brain vs. Left Brain (n.d.). Retrieved on: 5-16-2018. Retrieved from: http://www.funderstanding.com/brain/right-brain-vs-left-brain/.

be faster, meaning that random, intuitive thinking may be your communication style. Random thoughts that aren't logical and easily followed may not be a recipe for easy communication. Yet the synthesizing aspect of the right hemisphere will make communicating in groups an easier avenue of communication to enjoy.

If your right hemisphere is injured, your left hemisphere will provide logical reasoning that is sequential and easily followed. But you may struggle with the flexibility and adaptiveness and novelty of an exciting conversation. The effects of hemisphere production and compensation for injury all reveal themselves in peer communication.

Hemisphere Processing

Communication preferences will usually reveal hemisphere processing styles: who you choose to communicate with, how many communication partners you feel comfortable with (reflecting the right hemisphere's specialty of synthesizing and holistic processing), and the role in conversation you play. Do you feel more comfortable providing logical thoughts (a left hemisphere specialty, meaning the right hemisphere was injured) or do you find yourself coming up with random and subjective ideas (a right hemisphere specialty) that may have appeal and interest? Knowing which hemisphere style of communication and processing you specialize in is important and can direct your excellence as a communicator and indicate your success in peer relationships!

INSIGHT

Insight is the chance to make opportunity happen. It is the chance to make leaps in recovery, to find hidden chances within recovery and advances through personal realizations. Finding insight into a problem is finding that "aha" solution that uses a different type of problem-solving than what might be considered ordinary or logical. According to O'Brien,[53] "Insight is the sudden solution to a long-vexing problem, a sudden recognition of a new idea, or a sudden understanding of a complex situation…" (p. 1).

The way to encourage insight is not concentrating or fixating on a problem, however. According to O'Brien,[54] "To encourage insight, this means that we need to step back and let our minds wander or sleep on the problem. Insight cannot happen when our minds are constantly engaged" (p. 1).

Because insight can be a valuable recovery tool, it is worth it to use insight and discover the brain's potential. O'Brien[55] suggests that a person interested in fostering insight abilities should: "Engage in activities that encourage an open mind. Gather a wide base of knowledge, ask how

---

53   O'Brien (2017). Retrieved on 5-18-2018. Retrieved from: http://neuroscienceschool.com/2017/11/10insight-creative-problem-solving/.
54   O'Brien (2017). Retrieved on 5-18-2018. Retrieved from: http://neuroscienceschool.com/2017/11/10insight-creative-problem-solving/.
55   O'Brien (2017). Retrieved on 5-18-2018. Retrieved from: http://neuroscienceschool.com/2017/11/10insight-creative-problem-solving/.

you could do this differently, engage in a new hobby that uses completely different skills, or just generally relax and let your mind wander. Sleeping on the problem, meditating, or stepping away from it and concentrating on something else may help your unconscious mind to cultivate a… solution…" (p. 2).

Insight is a valuable skill to possess because of the effects of brain injury. According to ABIOS,[56] "Lack of insight or denial of difficulties or impairments can be a significant problem for some people after an acquired brain injury. A person may have limited or no awareness about their physical, cognitive, personality, or behavioral changes" (p. 1). This is why insight is so valuable in recovery and can be essential. A moment of inspiration causes a new recovery focus, or it can be the thoughts that come without focus—that come from your wandering mind. Either way, insight can bring you what you didn't know you needed.

Peer Experience: Insight

Head injury causes such a difficult situation with relation to awareness and insight into different problems. Recoveries often become so personally involving that insight that would help to overcome recovery problems is interrupted.

Concentrating focus to enable recovery can bring feelings of success and can bring the focus that the brain needs to learn and remember. Focus can bring the realization that skills need to be added to a recovery, but focus can also hide the insight and realization of how to get there.

Insight is a definite aspect of a healthy recovery. Different approaches must be used to find the different aspects which bring solutions to problems you cannot understand yet. Recognizing the usefulness of insight can mean the difference between a recovery that is realized or not.

INVESTIGATION

Head injury recovery requires an investigative approach to discovering success. Finding success with a head injury recovery requires introspection, performance research, and defining how you may need a change in your life. If you pursue this type of investigation in your recovery, you will undoubtedly see positive change.

Concentrating on being aware, asking questions, and being introspective during the therapy process can be essential to how you process and understand the therapy. Therapists may explain the importance of each exercise, leading you to prioritize different exercises because of how easy

---

56 ABIOS Acquired Brain Injury Outreach Service. Retrieved on 5-18-2018. Retrieved from: https://www.health.qld.gov.au/_data/assets/pdf_file/0037/3888576/insight_aware_fsw.pdf.

they are for you or how effective they are in terms of rehabilitation.

Performance research requires doing the therapy with intensity and recording any problems or unexpected results. It requires commitment toward repeating the exercises as best you can and incorporating the therapy into your life. Feeling rewarded after a time of therapy is one of the best feelings.

Finally, investigating and determining how you will define therapy—as a habit that can be engaged in once in a while or as a needed part of the day—will determine how you stick to it. Also investigating how easy you can make it fit into your life success will allow you to find a way to stick with it. Begin with therapy in the morning and get it out of the way, or wait until night to finish the day strong—just find the pattern of success that works for you.

> **Peer Experience with Investigation**
>
> **Investigating success is one of the most important aspects of recovery and rehabilitation. Not only is it important to be introspective; it is also important to achieve a level of performance and invest in that performance. It is important to determine how therapy will be defined in your life and how you feel success with it. Investigation can be one of the most beneficial aspects with which to approach recovery and how you discover the best of yourself.**

Johari Window

The Johari window is a communication model that improves awareness of communication needs and leadership opportunities. According to Communication Theory,[57] "It is necessary to improve self-awareness and personal development among individuals when they are in a group. The… window model is a convenient method used to achieve this task of understanding and enhancing communication between the members of a group. This model is also denoted as a feedback/ disclosure model of self-awareness. The Johari window is used to enhance the individual's perception of others. This model is based on two ideas—trust can be acquired by revealing information about you to others and learning yourselves from their feedbacks. Each person is represented by the Johari model through four quadrants or window panes…[each] signifies personal information, feelings, motivation and whether the information is known to oneself or others in four viewpoints" (p. 1-2). The Johari window shows what is known to self and others, and then what is not known to self or others.

These areas and windows will indicate the difficulty and awareness experienced when communicating with groups or even with individuals. A person denying their need for support will

---

57 Communication Theory (n.d). The Johari Window Model. Retrieved on: 5-18-2018. Retrieved from: https://www. Communicationtheory.org/the-johari-window-model/.

have a blind spot in their ability to communicate with a group. In the pane that is not known to self or others, teamwork becomes challenging.

The Johari window is a concept that can actually demonstrate what is going on with individual communication. In the box below, references to Harris[58] allow the understanding of how window concepts can apply to each survivor's situation. It can display whether personal disclosure is being useful to the communication process and how knowledge of self and others can influence the communication process.

Peer Experience: Johari Window

The Johari window can demonstrate the powerful ability of self-disclosure and the usefulness of communication or interpersonal restraint. Peer communication awareness can benefit from this model and demonstrate how denial can be a factor that works against an individual. There are communication labels that refer to communication as "secret, open, unknown, [and] blind." Can you think of any communication situations when you're communicating with these qualities? How someone who maybe doesn't know about your head injury or can detect your disabilities is essentially "sharing" your secret of your head injury until you tell them about it! The secret category reveals "secrets you know about yourself, but aren't comfortable sharing with others" (p. 3). Open communication refers to the communication that you "share easily with others about yourself" (p. 3) such as your favorite color or hobbies. The unknown category is "unknown to you or others" (p. 3). The blind category is when there are "things others can readily see about you that you are not aware of about yourself" (p. 3). Can you see how these communication categories can describe communication possibilities in a head injury?

J*UDGMENT*

The judgment we have toward our communication possibilities presents opportunities and constraints. It may be good to understand what types of communication will be successful to engage in when negatively approaching a conversation with the idea that "I will have difficulties communicating here." Expectations of difficulties that may never be experienced will negatively influence your experience before you even begin. The judgment of whether communication will be successful is dependent on who you communicate with and whether you take the opportunity to communicate.

Sharing a message with a communication partner is a gift. The choice of who we get to practice communication principles with is limitless. Anyone can choose to make a conversation go well and

---

58 Harris (2017). Johari Window: A Communication Tool to Improve Relationships. Retrieved from: https://youmemindbody.com/mental-health/Johari-Window. Retrieved on: 12-14-2019.

be accepting. Who you choose to communicate with or call your peers will influence the success you feel with communication; the peers you may go to a support group with or you find yourself hanging out with want to communicate with you.

They want to communicate and heal with you, just like your communication with them is healing. It is the act of communicating that brings healing from trauma. By communicating and relating, your brain is healing. By bringing other communication partners into your communication patterns, you influence your brain's ability to deal with trauma. The judgment of who is right to be your communication partner is an important step to help to heal trauma.

Comfort is brought by sharing an experience with someone. Regardless of the person you're communicating with, regardless of how you feel the communication is going, the act of communicating can be a healing act.

The true benefit of a communication is realizing healing is offered. The person who can tell their story heals from the trauma they have experienced. The experience of trauma may be a signal for the brain to reach out to others. You may find yourself drawn to reach out to someone and not know why. That is the magic of the brain knowing its internal needs; it wants to be rid of the trauma that is affecting it. Understanding the brain's unique sense of timing and needs can amount to a confusing set of behaviors and impulses, but make no judgment—the brain understands its needs and schedule of healing. It is waiting for you to help it heal.

Peer Experience: Judgment

The healing and communication possibilities offered by peers and those around us are relationships that can deal with the trauma that has been experienced. Each step toward another is one more step toward healing with better relationship skills.

The connections made will influence how a person operates and how a person finds themselves. Finding connection will influence better connections to ourselves. That changes the recovery picture of being able to interact with individual needs and circumstances. Your peers are around you. And healing is within you. Make no judgments—connection will enhance your recovery and build your ability to live with trauma.

*K*INDNESS

Kindness can turn a relationship around, bringing the aspects of respect and graciousness while interacting with your relationship partner. Connecting with your partner's needs and interacting with those needs are essential parts of kindness. According to Baines,[59] "…Happiest couples picked

---

59 Baines (n.d.). 8 Types of Kindness that Improve Any Relationship. Retrieved on: 5-21-18. Retrieved from http://www.beliefnet. com/love-family/relationships/ 8-tytpes-of-kindess-improve-any-…

up on cues for attention and gave it about 86 percent of the time. Couples who would go on to divorce only gave attention 33 percent of the time… Be kind by responding to your partner's need for attention. After all, everyone wants to be validated and noticed, especially by the person most important to them" (p. 1).

Kindness is not only choosing to interact with your relationship partner's needs; it is also about being present with the aspects of the relationship. Reflect on the 86 percent for the happiest couples compared to 33 percent of noticing attention cues for couples who were unhappy. Imagine if your partner's cues were noticed every time! The kindness would allow a better relationship!

Peer Experience: Kindness

The kindnesses that can define a relationship may be frustrating to someone who struggles with awareness. You may miss opportunities to be kind because of having to struggle so hard just to find yourself.

But if you can learn how to pay attention to your partner in the relationship, you can actually find ways that will add to the relationship. By focusing on how you will reinforce and support your partner's need for validation or reinforcement, opportunities will present themselves.

GAINING KNOWLEDGE

Gaining knowledge can be such an important aspect of learning peer relationships, yet the most frustrating realization about learning is that things must be forgotten to be remembered. According to the University of Glasgow,[60] "…Forgetting is a key part of learning" (p. 1).

Not only is forgetting essential for memory; it is also essential for the transfer of memories that will apply to new situations. According to the University of Glasgow,[61] "'Memory instability'— which prevents us from holding onto new memories—was key to the brain's ability to transfer experiences and skills to new situations. Memories that were stable, or complete, prevented knowledge transfer. In short, forgetting your experience is essential to being able to transfer skills from one job to another" (p. 1).

60 University of Glasgow (2015). Forgetting Is Key to Learning. Retrieved on: 5-21-2018. Retrieved from: http://www.gla.ac.uk/news/archiveofnews/2015/december/headline_437758_en.html.
61 University of Glasgow (2015). Forgetting Is Key to Learning. Retrieved on: 5-21-2018. Retrieved from: http://www.gla.ac.uk/news/archiveofnews/2015/december/headline_437758_en.html.

> **Peer Experience: Gaining Knowledge**
>
> **The frustrating complexities of relationships will likely mean that a lot of forgetting needs to be done to allow memory transfer and skill application—skills that apply to different situations. Every communication situation can be viewed as different, as separate skills based on status, gender, and many other complex variables. Regardless of the time it may take to remember the way to better communication, it is worthwhile for recovery from trauma and being able to transfer skills. Remember, every time you struggle with deciding what to do, or figuring out the next step in communication which you're sure you've done before, know that what you're forgetting is likely adding essential skills to your communication.**

LEADERSHIP

Healing from trauma and peer relationships takes leadership and directive ability as well as the intangibles that communicate it. According to Hasan,[62] "Irrespective of how you define a leader, he or she can prove to be a difference maker between success and failure. A good leader has…vision and knows how to turn…ideas into real-world success stories" (p. 1). It takes both long- and short-term goals, and the ability to persevere and monitor feedback to examine if that is what you want. Leadership is having the ability to motivate yourself and push yourself to the places you need to go.

Leadership relies on abilities that allow it to be carried out. According to Hasan,[63] "You will have to set a good example for others to follow. That is where your commitment, passion, empathy, honesty, and integrity come into play. Good communication skill and decision-making capabilities also play a vital role in success and failure of a leader… Innovation and creative thinking, as well as…vision…make a leader stand out" (p. 5).

Leadership is not only knowing how to lead or the places where you need to go; it is also knowing where you've been and being able to acknowledge that. If we are not able to be in touch with the experiences that have brought us here, denial enters the recovery situation. When denial is impacting the recovery of an individual, recovery is not representative of an individual's leadership situation. The brain is on its own schedule of healing and recovering from trauma. Many of your feelings will be representative of what the brain needs, but some of those options it sees may not be good for your recovery.

Short-term and long-term goals are one type of leadership method that will enable a progressive recovery. Peer communication and concepts may cause frustration, but what needs to be understood

---

62 Hasan (2017). Top 10 Leadership Qualities That Make Good Leaders. Retrieved on: 5-22-2018. Retrieved from: https://blog.taskque.com/characteristics-good-leaders/.

63 Hasan (2017). Top 10 Leadership Qualities That Make Good Leaders. Retrieved on: 5-22-2018. Retrieved from: https://blog.taskque.com/characteristics-good-leaders/.

are the benefits over the pain and difficulty of finding success with those peer relationships.

The brain needs your leadership to live an enhanced life. The brain will give you feedback of the successes, but it is waiting for the leadership in you to interpret the successes. Maybe you had a long night, which is interfering with the processing speed that you rely on to interact with your peers. The leader in you has just learned something. When you decide to understand the results of fatigue meaning a difficulty interacting with peers, the leader within will understand and realize that you experience better communication when well rested. Leadership means planning for better sleep or reduced interactions after a night with no sleep. Leadership: it's the force behind recoveries.

Peer Experience: Leadership

Leadership relies on being the best of who you truly are. Finding the best aspects of yourself and leading with those gifts that we each have make leadership situations.

Maybe it's your anger that moves you and you're wondering how you can make that proactively work for your recovery. It does move you, and you connect with it, so find success using anger in your rehabilitation exercises. Find the connection between your anger and recovery and follow it.

Leadership is not only finding leadership activities; it's also about doing the small intangibles that no one ever notices. Find the attention to detail, do the hard stuff, and before long, your leadership will define you.

LOVE

The draw of the word *love* can mean different things to many people. Love can fill the heart of a person who finds they want that connection. The chemicals, body reactions, and changes in thinking can easily reinforce this feeling of love. Love has been a motivating factor that has rewarded humanity in primitive times. According to Edwards,[64] "We know that primitive areas of the brain are involved in romantic love…and that these areas light up on brain scans when talking about a loved one. These areas can stay lit up for a long time for some couples" (p. 2).

The reward of love doesn't stop there. Love also changes thoughts and figuring. The reward system being activated consists of dopamine.[65] "Being love-struck also releases high levels of dopamine, a chemical that gets the reward system going…helping to make love a pleasurable experience similar to the euphoria associated with the use of cocaine or alcohol" (p. 2).

---

64 Edwards (n.d.). Love and the Brain. Retrieved on 5-22-2018. Retrieved from: http://neuro.hms.harvard.edu/harvard-mahoney-neuroscience-institute/brain-newsletter/ and…

65 Edwards (n.d.). Love and the Brain. Retrieved on 5-22-2018. Retrieved from: http://neuro.hms.harvard.edu/harvard-mahoney-neuroscience-institute/brain-newsletter/ and…

The positive rewards of dopamine change the person who experiences it.[66] "In addition to the positive feelings romance brings, love also deactivates the neural pathway responsible for negative emotions, such as fear and social judgment" (p. 3).

Reward systems and the mind become accustomed to the reward of love, and partners change their perspectives, with[67] "…an inevitable change over time from passionate love to what is typically called compassionate love—love that is deep but not as euphoric as that experienced during the early stages of romance" (p. 3).

Love becomes a responsibility to keep up or fall out of. It is a nurturing part of relationships that gives a reward and has been a primary driver of humanity. The choice to love is individual, yet the feelings of love bringing reward are universal.

Peer Experience: Love

The choice of love and the dream of it can move mountains. The feelings of love are so powerful that they change lives and may be what a person spends many of their years searching for.

When love is found, however, there will be a choice to try to continue the passion of the relationship or to find a deeper area of compassion within the love. Love is a gift and can contain the feelings of addiction, and until it is realistically approached, love may seem uncontrollable and fleeting or it can be brought consistent attention.

MEDITATION

Meditation is a life- and potential-changing exercise. According to Gladding,[68] "Sitting [and concentrating on breathing] every day, for at least 15-20 minutes, makes a huge difference in how you approach life, how personally you take things and how you interact with others. It enhances compassion, allows you to see things more clearly (including yourself) and creates a sense of calm and centeredness that is indescribable" (p. 1).

The part of the brain meditation enhances is the[69] "lateral prefrontal cortex…the part of the brain that allows you to look at things from a more rational, logical, and balanced perspective… we'll call it the **Assessment Center.** It is involved in modulating emotional responses (originating from the fear center of the brain), overriding automatic behaviors/habits, and decreasing the brain's

---

66 Edwards (n.d.). Love and the Brain. Retrieved on 5-22-2018. Retrieved from: http://neuro.hms.harvard.edu/harvard-mahoney-neuroscience-institute/brain-newsletter/ and…

67 Edwards (n.d.). Love and the Brain. Retrieved on 5-22-2018. Retrieved from: http://neuro.hms.harvard.edu/harvard-mahoney-neuroscience-institute/brain-newsletter/ and…

68 Gladding (2013). This Is Your Brain on Meditation. Retrieved on: 5-22-18. Retrieved from: https://www.psychologytoday.com/us/blog/use-your-mind-change-your-brain/201305/is-y…

69 Gladding (2013). This Is Your Brain on Meditation. Retrieved on: 5-22-18. Retrieved from: https://www.psychologytoday.com/us/blog/use-your-mind-change-your-brain/201305/is-y…

tendency to take things personally…" (p. 1).

Another part of the brain affected by meditation is the medial prefrontal cortex. "{It] is the part of the brain that constantly references back to you, your perspective and experiences. Many call this the **Me Center** of the brain because it processes information related to you, inferring other people's state of mind or feeling empathy for others…call it the Self-Referencing Center" (p. 1).

The medial prefrontal cortex has two sections[70]—one part is "…involved in processing related to you and people that you view as *similar* to you" (p. 1). The next part, according to Gladding,[71] is involved in "processing information related to people who you perceive as being *dissimilar* from you. This very important part of the brain is involved in feeling empathy…" (p. 1).

Meditating is a crucial aspect of enhancing empathy.[72] "[The connections established] explain why meditation enhances empathy…the end result is that we are more able to put ourselves in another person's shoes…increasing empathy and compassion for everyone" (p. 3). Meditation is a reality-enhancing practice. According to Gladding,[73] "The very real rewards gained from meditation combine to form a compelling argument for developing and/or maintaining a daily practice... Even if it's only 15 minutes, it will keep those newly formed connections strong and the unhelpful ones of the past at bay" (p. 4). Meditation can enhance your social brain more than you can imagine. Why aren't you doing it?

Peer Experience: Meditation

Enhancing perspectives on reality and encouraging empathy are just the beginning argument to be made to find meditation as an aspect of improving social skills. Stopping bad habits, encouraging higher processing, and encouraging a sense of more complete communication, meditation offers many reasons to concentrate on your breathing.

MINDFULNESS

Mindfulness is a novel approach to understanding recovery needs and feelings. Acceptance is the major emphasis that makes mindfulness an outstanding recovery tool. Being aware of different impulses and realizing they are just reactions will enhance recovery. It turns struggling to be accepted by a peer group into accepting that the peer group is struggling with anxiety, which is discouraging rapport.

---

70   Gladding (2013). This Is Your Brain on Meditation. Retrieved on: 5-22-18. Retrieved from: https://www.psychologytoday.com/us/blog/use-your-mind-change-your-brain/201305/is-y...

71   Gladding (2013). This Is Your Brain on Meditation. Retrieved on: 5-22-18. Retrieved from: https://www.psychologytoday.com/us/blog/use-your-mind-change-your-brain/201305/is-y...

72   Gladding (2013). This Is Your Brain on Meditation. Retrieved on: 5-22-18. Retrieved from: https://www.psychologytoday.com/us/blog/use-your-mind-change-your-brain/201305/is-y...

73   Gladding (2013). This Is Your Brain on Meditation. Retrieved on: 5-22-18. Retrieved from: https://www.psychologytoday.com/us/blog/use-your-mind-change-your-brain/201305/is-y...

Mindfulness is what encourages true responses to emerge from recovery. According to Hayes[74], "…'Mindfulness' has been used to refer to a psychological state of awareness. The practices that promote this awareness [are] a mode of processing information and a character trait" (p. 2).

Exercises and routines do encourage mindfulness.[75] "Several disciplines and practices cultivate mindfulness… most of the literature…developed through mindfulness meditation—those self-regulation practices on training attention and awareness to bring mental processes under greater voluntary control and…foster general well-being and development [of] calmness, clarity, and concentration" (p. 2-3).

Mindfulness meditation deals with focusing on the breath while remaining acutely aware. Higher cognitive abilities and processing are accessed with reliance on meditation and calming acceptance. Accepting feelings that come into awareness and letting them go because you realize they are just feelings, nothing more or less, allows you to enjoy certain benefits. Mindfulness offers benefits like[76] "reduced rumination, stress reduction, Boosts to memory, focus, less emotional reactivity, more cognitive flexibility, [and] relationship satisfaction" (p. 3-5).

Being present with the situation and attentive to non-judgmental feelings allows mindfulness to result in proactivity to the situation. The benefits of mindfulness for the brain are exceptional. Relationships especially benefit.[77] "A person's ability to be mindful can help predict relationship satisfaction—the ability to respond well to relationship stress and the skill in communicating one's emotions to a partner" (p. 4).

Peer Experience: Mindfulness

One of the benefits of mindfulness is relationship success. Adding focus and reducing rumination while increasing non-judgment and acceptance influences relationship interaction and being present for your partner.

Mindfulness adds another dimension to relationships. It brings acceptance of self into a relationship and allows a level of engagement. Opportunities reveal themselves when accepting and focusing on delivering a higher level of processing.

---

74   Hayes (2012). What are the Benefits of Mindfulness. Retrieved on: 5-23-18. Retrieved from: http://www.apa.org/monitor /2012-08/ce-corner.aspx

75   Hayes (2012). What are the Benefits of Mindfulness. Retrieved on: 5-23-18. Retrieved from: http://www.apa.org/monitor /2012-08/ce-corner.aspx

76   Hayes (2012). What Are the Benefits of Mindfulness. Retrieved on: 5-23-18. Retrieved from: http://www.apa.org/monitor /2012-08/ce-corner.aspx.

77   Hayes (2012). What Are the Benefits of Mindfulness. Retrieved on: 5-23-18. Retrieved from: http://www.apa.org/monitor /2012-08/ce-corner.aspx.

Needs of a Relationship

Relationships have needs that each partner presents. All relationships are different, yet they do have many of the same components. According to Psychology Today,[78] "Successful couples make their relationships work" (p. 1). Using skills for a relationship which can help a person heal from trauma brings a **PEACEFUL** approach to engaging in relationships while healing trauma."

Politeness[79]—"Even if you're offended…keep your anger in check. As soon as the opportunity arises to discuss what happened, take it. You don't want to hold on to anything you don't need to" (p. 1) Knowing the needs of the relationship and being polite are essential.

Emotional support[80]—"This may be the single most valuable component in a relationship. Having someone in your corner while you navigate through…is the highest order" (p. 1).

Accountability[81]—"If you screw up, admit it and apologize if it's called for. Keep your word and know that trust is something that is continually earned" (p. 1).

Compliment[82]—"Kind words, given at the right time, are fuel for the future to those who are fortunate to receive them. Giving compliments to the one you love helps you to keep connected" (p. 1).

Engage your partner with questions[83]—"Show interest in what your other half is doing by asking about what's going on in his or her life and how he or she is feeling about things. This will create an opportunity to keep your emotions balanced" (p. 1).

Future planning and present living[84]—"Goals are important to your overall happiness, and having a contingency plan in case of an emergency will allow you to enjoy your time together more thoroughly" (p. 1).

Understanding another person's feelings[85]—"Making a joke at someone else's expense always stings the other person. Name calling is downright insulting. If you engage in this dangerous game, stop while you still have someone to play with" (p. 1).

Loving requirements[86]— "Stay connected physically. Holding hands, exchanging foot rubs,

---

78 Psychology Today (2012). 10 Steps to a Closer Relationship. Retrieved on 5-23-2018. Retrieved from: https://www.psychology-today.com/us/blog/emotional-fitness/20111/10-steps-closer-relati…

79 Psychology Today (2012). 10 Steps to a Closer Relationship. Retrieved on 5-23-2018. Retrieved from: https://www.psychology-today.com/us/blog/emotional-fitness/20111/10-steps-closer-relati…

80 Psychology Today (2012). 10 Steps to a Closer Relationship. Retrieved on 5-23-2018. Retrieved from: https://www.psychology-today.com/us/blog/emotional-fitness/20111/10-steps-closer-relati…

81 Psychology Today (2012). 10 Steps to a Closer Relationship. Retrieved on 5-23-2018. Retrieved from: https://www.psychology-today.com/us/blog/emotional-fitness/20111/10-steps-closer-relati…

82 Psychology Today (2012). 10 Steps to a Closer Relationship. Retrieved on 5-23-2018. Retrieved from: https://www.psychology-today.com/us/blog/emotional-fitness/20111/10-steps-closer-relati…

83 Psychology Today (2012). 10 Steps to a Closer Relationship. Retrieved on 5-23-2018. Retrieved from: https://www.psychology-today.com/us/blog/emotional-fitness/20111/10-steps-closer-relati…

84 Psychology Today (2012). 10 Steps to a Closer Relationship. Retrieved on 5-23-2018. Retrieved from: https://www.psychology-today.com/us/blog/emotional-fitness/20111/10-steps-closer-relati…

85 Psychology Today (2012). 10 Steps to a Closer Relationship. Retrieved on 5-23-2018. Retrieved from: https://www.psychology-today.com/us/blog/emotional-fitness/20111/10-steps-closer-relati…

86 Psychology Today (2012). 10 Steps to a Closer Relationship. Retrieved on 5-23-2018. Retrieved from: https://www.psychology-today.com/us/blog/emotional-fitness/20111/10-steps-closer-relati…

the feel of your partner's hand touching your back as you pass each other in the hallway—these moments are as important as making love. One day they will be more important" (p. 1). The needs of a relationship need to be considered and adapted for your partner.

Peer Experience: Needs of a Relationship

Resolving trauma with relationships can be the most PEACEFUL way to deal with recovery and finding who you truly are. The aspects of relationships that need to be satisfied are all indicated by the acronym PEACEFUL. How many of the skills of the PEACEFUL acronym do you use already? Finding the most PEACEFUL way to overcome your trauma by engaging in relationship skills can be the answer to your health!

NEUROPLASTICITY

Neuroplasticity is the life-changing, recovery-changing brain concept enabling new skills and responsibilities. There are certain aspects that influence brain change. According to Hampton,[87] "Neuroplasticity makes your brain extremely resilient and is the process by which all learning takes place in your brain, such as playing a musical instrument or mastering a different language… Neuroplasticity has far-reaching implications and possibilities for almost every aspect of human life and culture from education to medicine" (p. 3).

Brain change is especially important for new learning or skills, such as learning the crucial aspects of socialization and interaction. The top three aspects that influence neuroplasticity and brain change follow:[88]

1. **"Change is mostly limited to those situations in which the brain is in the mood for it.** If you are alert, on the ball, engaged, motivated, ready for action, the brain releases the neurochemicals necessary to enable brain change. When disengaged, inattentive, distracted, or doing something without thinking that requires no real effort, your neuroplastic switches are 'off.'

2. **The harder you try, the more you're motivated, the more alert you are, and the better (or worse) the potential outcome, the higher the brain change.** If you're intensely focused on the task and really trying to master something for an important reason, the change experienced will be greater.

---

87 Hampton (n.d). Neuroplasticity: The 10 Fundamentals of Rewiring Your Brain—Reset me. Retrieved on: 5-22-2018. Retrieved from: http://reset.me/story/neuroplasticity-the-10-fundamentals-of-rewiring-your-brain/.

88 Hampton (n.d). Neuroplasticity: The 10 Fundamentals of Rewiring Your Brain—Reset me. Retrieved on: 5-22-2018. Retrieved from: http://reset.me/story/neuroplasticity-the-10-fundamentals-of-rewiring-your-brain/.

3. **What actually changes in the brain are the strengths of the connections of neurons that are engaged together, moment by moment, in time.** The more something is practiced, the more connections are changed and made to include all elements of the experience (sensory, info, movement, cognitive patterns). You can think of it like a 'master controller' being formed for that particular behavior, which allows it to be performed with remarkable facility and reliability over time" (p. 4).

Peer Experience: Neuroplasticity

Social learning has the potential to carry many frustrations and learning impediments because of disability. Yet, by remaining motivated and aware, emphasizing the potential benefits of socialization, and the more effort put into practice, the better chance you have at turning a difficult concept to learn to become a healing concept that overcomes trauma. The brain is ready to learn; the truth of every learning situation is how ready you are to allow the brain to change. Find the motivation to learn the skills you need to learn, spend the time practicing the skills you need to remember, and be the example of neuroplasticity that your brain is representative of.

OPTIMISM

The optimism that each relationship partner has about their relationship may be a demonstration of resistance or inability to change. According to Stadtmiller,[89] "There is a scientific name for my thinking, it turns out, called 'optimism bias.' Scientists estimate that 80 percent of people exhibit the behavior, which…isn't doing them any favors when it comes to relationships" (p. 2).

Optimism is needed in recovery; the tint of positivity needs to influence recovery expectations. The best thinking depends on it. Thought agility and direction are contingent upon positivity. Yet thoughts influenced by denial are not the nimblest that take us to better recovery outcomes. According to Stadtmiller,[90] an "…incredibly illuminating…study…followed 501…couples over the course of four years: All…reported…themselves as 'highly optimistic' about their coupling were more likely to report dissatisfaction later on" (p. 2).

The truth hidden within optimism is for couples needing to accept responsibility. Stadtmiller[91] "…advised…individuals 'to realize their strengths and weakness and calibrate their standards accordingly'—and that high expectations could be as toxic as poor communication" (p. 2).

---

89   Stadtmiller (2016). Forget Optimism: Choose Realism Instead. Retrieved on: 5-22-2018. Retrieved from: https://www.thecut.com/2016/11/is-too-much-optimism-in-relationships -a-bad-thing.html.

90   Stadtmiller (2016) Forget Optimism: Choose Realism Instead. Retrieved on:5-22-2018. Retrieved from: https://www.thecut.com/2016/11/is-too-much-optimism-in-relationships -a-bad-thing.html.

91   Stadtmiller (2016) Forget Optimism: Choose Realism Instead. Retrieved on:5-22-2018. Retrieved from: https://www.thecut.com/2016/11/is-too-much-optimism-in-relationships -a-bad-thing.html.

Find the acceptance within yourself and your relationship expectations. Don't encumber yourself with expectations that will hurt your relationship.

Peer Experience: Optimism

The reality of accepting the health of your relationship mirrors how your relationship skills can enable change. By trying to find the best skills to enable the best relationship, you can realize empowerment from the predisposition for acceptance and realism. It can change relationships and encourage happiness.

Find the motivation to change and become the best relationship partner by concentrating on your strengths. Enable your best relationship with acceptance and love of reality.

OXYTOCIN

Oxytocin is one of the chemicals that can enhance and lead relationships. According to Psychology Today,[92] "Oxytocin is a powerful hormone that acts as a neurotransmitter in the brain. It regulates social interaction…empathy, [and] generosity… When we hug or kiss a loved one, oxytocin levels increase; hence, oxytocin is often called 'the love hormone'…plays a huge role in pair bonding. Oxytocin is the hormone that underlies trust. It is also an antidote to depressive feelings" (p. 1).

Peer Experience: Oxytocin

The trust within a relationship that influences bonding. The hugs you give to your close friend that bring trust and understanding and predispose you to act with generosity toward each other are an effect of the hormone oxytocin. Oxytocin can even mediate depressive feelings, showing that the bonds of relationships are amazing.

Even the social norm of touch is meant to elicit and emphasize the effects of oxytocin. A handshake over a business deal is meant to signify the establishment of a trusting relationship between business partners; a hug between family members is meant to bring feelings of closeness. Oxytocin's powerful effects can come to be used for relationships that you want to renew or bring life to.

PASSION

Passion is the fuel for interest of others. Passion gives freedom to the internal drives and interests that can be attractive in a peer situation. Even more, passion is exactly where the brain needs to be.

---

92   Psychology Today (n.d.). https://www.psychologytoday.com/us/basics/oxytocin.

According to Black,[93] "Passion brings energy. Passion helps create change and movement. Passion creates a positive environment. Passion ignites others. Passion drives others. Passion drives vision. Passion increases influence. Passion brings opportunity and opens the door to success..." (p. 1).

Peer Experience: Passion

Passion opens the mind to possibility and influences the possibilities of energy manifesting into positive production. Following your passion around your peers creates the leadership which peers can follow. Passion is the flame that ignites interests and burns with desire. The changes that passion creates in the brain and the opportunities following a passion lead to success.

PREMACK PRINCIPLE

The hectic and disagreeable schedule of recovery and rehabilitation gets much calmer and more enjoyable when using the Premack Principle. A principle that can carry both rehabilitation and peer interaction to success, the Premack Principle is[94] "using a high probability behavior...to reinforce a low probability behavior..." (p. 1).

This changes an infrequent, disagreeable event into a favorite practice that is repeated often and made meaningful. By pairing the disagreeable event (possibly doing therapy exercises) with an enjoyable event (watching your favorite TV program), you allow yourself to do therapy every night your favorite program is on!

Accessing principles that make neuroplasticity a driving force behind brain change, the Premack Principle is a driving force behind learning and enjoyable practice. It can also be used to enhance peer interactions. By paying attention to another peer's favorite activities and then making them a part of your schedule, you encourage their associations and enjoyment of the activity to be paired with you. Before long, you can find yourself in a situation that encourages a peer relationship!

---

93   Black (n.d). The Benefits of Passion. Retrieved on: 5-23-2018. Retrieved from: http://danblackonleadership.info/archives/594.

94   Robert S. Premack Principle: Definition & Example. Retrieved on 5-21-2018. Retrieved from: https://study.com/academy/lesson/premack-principle-defintion-example.html.

Peer Experience: Premack Principle

The concept of an enjoyable meeting or date revolves around the Premack Principle. Successful rehabilitation and recovery principles benefit from the use of the Premack Principle as well. By placing the television remote control by the phone, you access and pair the draw of one of your favorite forms of entertainment (watching TV) with a challenging recovery principle of healing from trauma. You decide that before you get to watch TV, you must call a friend and communicate. Before long, you are enjoying your communication opportunities just like how you remember you once enjoyed television! When your communication partner learns your favorite TV program is their favorite program, you might decide to watch it together! The Premack Principle has just worked for you!

QUESTION OF CALLING

After a traumatic experience like a head injury, the question that can be life-defining—finding a calling, or something that you feel strongly about investing in and completing as a life mission—can be answered by answering these seven questions to discover your calling:[95]

1. What is your message to the world?
2. What kind of legacy do you want to leave?
3. What doesn't feel like work to you?
4. What did you imagine doing when you were a kid?
5. Who is doing your dream job? And what exactly is that job?
6. What are you most passionate about?
7. What work would you never do again no matter how much you were paid? (p. 2-3)

Peer Experience: Question of Calling

The question of calling allows a feeling of belonging that is not easily achieved in other ways. By finding a directive that predisposes you to find and believe in life more than avoiding trauma, a question of calling allows you to discover the meaning in life and begin to unearth it. If your calling speaks to you clearly enough, the trauma you experienced may be overtaken by the calling you find as your mission to fulfill.

---

95   7 Questions to Help You Discover Your Life's Calling. (2015).

Question Thinking

The questions that come up in recovery are the questions that can change our life.[96] "The questions we ask ourselves on a daily basis could very well be the most critical and important factors that determine our ongoing success, happiness, and fulfillment in life" (p. 1). The questions that we ask ourselves expose the limited view of reality that we see. Each question we ask exposes directions and approaches to different recovery situations. According to Sicinski,[97] "…questions are mysterious blessings, yet at the same time, they can be deadly precursors to a life of misery and heartache…questioning patterns that will either lead us to a life of fulfillment or a life of unrealized potential" (p. 2).

Do you find that your questions are setting you up to be reactive or to feel at a loss? That may be a clue that the questions you are finding within yourself need to be examined, and a different type of questioning be participated in. Sicinski[98] reports, "Our questions help alter the perspective of the world around us. These questions essentially color how we view ourselves, others, objects, events, and circumstances in ways that help us see things in a new light and from a unique and different angle" (p. 3).

The questions you find in your life that will affect you and the reality you see are going to alter your responses and change the proactivity and leadership you feel you can use. The questions you will find within yourself are the questions that will often determine your recovery or the extent of your relationship with your peer that will heal your trauma. Awareness of your questions and the responses to those questions are the words, ideas, and applications that will lead your recovery.

Peer Experience: Question Thinking

The questions that truly impact us are the ones we ask after an unsatisfying performance or failure. Yet the real questions that I want you to ask yourself, or wait to respond to, are the questions that will encourage you with your relationships and ability. The questions that have reflected my reality and recovery direction were once, "What is wrong with me that no one likes me?" but it has changed to, "Is this new friend going to spend enough time to get to know me and appreciate me for who I am?" Completely different perspectives encourage completely different actions and responses.

---

96 Sicinski (n.d.). How To Get What You Want Faster Through Asking Better Questions. Retrieved on: 5-21-2018. Retrieved from: https://blog.iqmatrix.com/better-questions.

97 Sicinski (n.d.). How To Get What You Want Faster Through Asking Better Questions. Retrieved on: 5-21-2018. Retrieved from: https://blog.iqmatrix.com/better-questions.

98 Sicinski (n.d.). How To Get What You Want Faster Through Asking Better Questions. Retrieved on: 5-21-2018. Retrieved from: https://blog.iqmatrix.com/better-questions.

Relationship Hygiene

Many people enter a relationship with another having different ideas about what the relationship will provide for them. According to Goldsmith,[99] "A relationship cannot survive on its own. It needs the care and nurturing of two adults, giving to each other in a way that creates a mutually beneficial connection" (p. 1). Becoming aware of each other's expectations and providing for them is what relationship hygiene is all about. The Five Love Languages gives an amazing description of how to practice relationship hygiene. Each exercise it contains **TAGS-U** as a great relationship partner.

Touch—Touch is a powerful language that doesn't have to be heard. According to Kilpatrick,[100] "Physical touch is a powerful communicator" (p. 2).

Affirmations[101]—"Saying 'I love you,' giving compliments, and making positive statements about your loved one is one way of showing love" (p. 1).

Gifts—Gifts are an exchange of the generosity of the heart. According to Kilpatrick,[102] "A visual symbol of affection, gift giving is fundamental to love" (p. 2).

Service [and]—according to Kilpatrick,[103] "…performing thoughtful gestures that you know will please…" (p. 1).

Understanding the need for quality time, for quality relating and appreciating, is a very important love language.[104] "…spend time…hours or days in proximity…practice listening by giving…your undivided attention, not interrupting, making eye contact, and asking questions for clarity…" (p. 2).

By completing the needs and requirements of a relationship, the hygiene or upkeep of a relationship is provided. The needs of a relationship are provided for and delivered. Relationship hygiene allows a stronger establishment of a relationship and an amazing way to provide for a relationship.

---

99   Goldsmith (n.d.). 10 Things Your Relationship Needs to Thrive. Retrieved on: 5-22-2018. Retrieved from: https://www.psychologytoday.com/us/blog/emotional fitness/201303/10-things-your-relati…

100 Kilpatrick (n.d.). What Are the 5 Love Languages? Retrieved 5-30-2018. Retrieved from: https://everydaylife.com/love-languages-5533438.html.

101 Kilpatrick (n.d.). What Are the 5 Love Languages? Retrieved 5-30-2018. Retrieved from: https://everydaylife.com/love-languages-5533438.html.

102 Kilpatrick (n.d.). What Are the 5 Love Languages? Retrieved 5-30-2018. Retrieved from: https://everydaylife.com/love-languages-5533438.html.

103 Kilpatrick (n.d.). What Are the 5 Love Languages? Retrieved 5-30-2018. Retrieved from: https://everydaylife.com/love-languages-5533438.html.

104 Kilpatrick (n.d.). What Are the 5 Love Languages? Retrieved 5-30-2018. Retrieved from: https://everydaylife.com/love-languages-5533438.html.

Peer Experience: Relationship Hygiene

The maintenance of a relationship can get to be so complex that many may become overwhelmed by the idea of a relationship. But by simplifying relationship hygiene to an acronym, the idea of a relationship becomes much easier. A relationship can be difficult with trauma, yet when looked at with confidence and ability, it becomes easier.

Relationships are for all to enjoy. By engaging in one, you are showing that now is your time, that you can be the partner a relationship needs. Go and be the one who someone needs and enjoys.

RENEWAL STRATEGY

The strategy that motivates the brain to recover is a renewal strategy. Using the renewal strategy is indicative of finding the best of opportunities for healing and recovering from head injury. It relies on four aspects: **P**erspective, **A**utonomy, **C**onnectedness, and **T**onal. By using the renewal strategy, you are making a **PACT** with your recovery success! The **PACT** of success begins with:

Perspective—Your frame of mind enables the brain to feel and work at its best. According to Hampton,[105] "…when people consciously practice gratitude, they get a surge of rewarding neurotransmitters, like dopamine, and experience a general alerting and brightening of the mind, probably correlated with more of the neurochemical norepinephrine" (p. 2).

Autonomy—Autonomy is freeing your mind with the challenges in learning you take. According to Sharecare,[106] "To stay sharp as a whip, continue to challenge your brain on a daily basis" (p. 3).

Connectedness—Connection to your peers is healing for traumatic experiences and is a basic need for the brain. According to Smith,[107] "…we also have a basic need to belong in a group and form relationships" (p. 3).

Tonal—Connecting to health with exercise is important in the aspect of renewal. According to Schmitt,[108] "Before we can see the benefits exercise has on the brain, we should understand the two categories of exercise. Aerobic exercise is exercise you can do at a 'conversation' pace, like long distance running or any exercise lasting longer than 20-30 minutes…anaerobic exercise that taxes you to the point where you have to stop and catch your breath. These are very quick, maximal effort exercises such as sprinting, high-intensity interval training (HIIT), and Olympic lifts…. These categories of exercise have a very different but very positive effect on your brain" (p. 1).

---

105 Hampton (2017). How Your Thoughts Change Your Brain, Cells, and Genes. Retrieved on 5-26-2018. Retrieved from: https://www.huffingtonpost.com/debbie-hampton/how-your-thoughts-change-your-brain-c...

106 Sharecare (n.d.). Retrieved on: 5-26-2018. Retrieved from: https://www.sharecare.com/health/brain/learning-impact-on-the-brain.

107 Smith (2013). Social Connection Makes a Better Brain. Retrieved on: 5-26-2018. Retrieved from: https://www.theatlantic .com/health/archive/2013/10/social-connection-makes-a-better-brai…

108 Schmitt (n.d.). http://thefactorytraining.com/benefits-of-aerobic-and-anaerobic-exercise-on-the-brain/.

Peer Experience: Renewal Strategy

Taking the chance to renew the brain with the aspects of the renewal strategy means that by participating in the strategy, you also participate in improving your recovery. Making a PACT with recovery success by using the renewal strategy is easy to see.

The gratitude that enables better brain response pairs with the learning that is encouraged to keep the brain sharp. Communication satisfies an aspect of human needs and trauma recovery, while physical exercise enables benefits to the brain and positive effects to transform recovery. The PACT that is made by using the renewal strategy is an important aspect of keeping the brain in a state of readiness for healing.

S*ELF*

The self that we develop can encourage relationships, but it is the self we learn to take care of that encourages relational awareness and readiness. According to Mackler,[109] "Many people don't treat themselves very well. They break promises to themselves, eat poorly, don't get enough sleep, are self-critical or fail to take good care of their bodies. In fact, if most people treated others the way they treat themselves, they wouldn't have many friends!" (p. 1).

If we don't value the connection with ourselves enough, there may be a predisposition to not deliver the attention and caring, or invest in a relationship that a partner would deserve. According to Mackler,[110] "A great technique for treating yourself better is by developing your Inner Nurturing Parent. Imagine you had a little child in your care. You'd make every effort to keep her healthy and safe; to love and support her, to be forgiving of her mistakes, her inevitable slips; and to let her know how precious and important she is. That's what a loving parent does. Only, in this case, you're the parent and the child…" (p. 1).

Recommendations for self-care:[111] "…set healthy boundaries with others. Let people know what you want and don't want" (p. 2). Another bit of advice for care of self, according to Mackler,[112] is "Become your advocate…someone is disrespectful or hurtful to you, speak up…" (p. 2). A third suggestion for self-care[113] is "Believe in yourself… A nurturing parent would highlight your uniqueness, tell you how special you are, encourage you to build on your strengths, and support you

109 Mackler (2011). 7 Steps to Nurturing Your Inner Self. Retrieved on: 5-26-2018. Retrieved from: https://www.huffingtonpost.com/lauren-mackler/os-your-inner-child-under_b_710499.html.

110 Mackler (2011). 7 Steps to Nurturing Your Inner Self. Retrieved on: 5-26-2018. Retrieved from: https://www.huffingtonpost.com/lauren-mackler/os-your-inner-child-under_b_710499.html.

111 Mackler (2011). 7 Steps to Nurturing Your Inner Self. Retrieved on: 5-26-2018. Retrieved from: https://www.huffingtonpost.com/lauren-mackler/os-your-inner-child-under_b_710499.html.

112 Mackler (2011). 7 Steps to Nurturing Your Inner Self. Retrieved on: 5-26-2018. Retrieved from: https://www.huffingtonpost.com/lauren-mackler/os-your-inner-child-under_b_710499.html.

113 Mackler (2011). 7 Steps to Nurturing Your Inner Self. Retrieved on: 5-26-2018. Retrieved from: https://www.huffingtonpost.com/lauren-mackler/os-your-inner-child-under_b_710499.html.

in a loving, nonjudgmental way. A nurturing parent says, 'You can do it. I believe in you.' Become your strongest supporter, coach, and cheerleader" (p. 2). And finally,[114] "…Be compassionate with yourself. Have compassion for your humanity and your flaws. You're human and you're going to make mistakes. Look at yourself through the eyes of a loving parent; don't punish or criticize yourself. Reassure yourself. Comfort yourself. Accept yourself unconditionally. And show the same compassion for your own parents and others, because they, too, are human" (p. 2).

How you take yourself will wire your brain to understand how you should treat others and the level of expectations you should have about treating others.

Peer Experience: Self

How we treat ourselves can be a model for how we need to treat others. Understanding that the treatment of ourselves is a model for the success of our relationships can bring attention to the aspects of how we treat ourselves. There is no better way to understand the need for patience for a partner who is struggling in a relationship than when you find yourself responding to your struggling and responding with nurturing reassurance.

Life success comes from practice. And there's no better practice for others than how you take care of yourself.

STRESS

Stress can be a limiting factor during a head injury, with negative effects for those experiencing it. According to Stupart,[115] "…stress can have wide-ranging effects on emotion, mood, and behavior. Stress affects both…physical and mental functioning…" (p. 2).

The stresses experienced by trying to fit in with a new peer group influence to heal the trauma that has been experienced. Common stressors[116] are "peer pressure, interpersonal pressure, [and] lack of support system" (p. 2), which all add to a stressful situation.

These common stressors point to the importance of peer acceptance to an individual recovering from trauma.

Stress levels may increase as you try to find belonging and acceptance. The most crucial aspect of peer relationships is that it is not how you are trying to make your peers like you; your peers accept you because they are your peers. Support groups are essential in finding peer support. Recovering from trauma using peer relationships is the life experience you share. You may feel

---

114 Mackler (2011). 7 Steps to Nurturing Your Inner Self. Retrieved on: 5-26-2018. Retrieved from: https://www.huffingtonpost.com/lauren-mackler/os-your-inner-child-under_b_710499.html.

115 Stupart (2018). Stress Affects College Students' Performance. Retrieved on: 5-26-2018. Retrieved from: https://owlcation.com/academia/College-Life-The-Effects-of-Stress-on-Academic-Perform…

116 Stupart (2018). Stress Affects College Students' Performance. Retrieved on: 5-26-2018. Retrieved from: https://owlcation.com/academia/College-Life-The-Effects-of-Stress-on-Academic-Perform…

unease when you are participating in the support groups, and you might enjoy just being silent and listening unless others invite you to talk.

Personal stress reactions, according to Stupart,[117] range from "frequent headaches, tremors, trembling of lips, neck and back pains, nervous habits, e.g., fidgeting, rapid or mumbled speech, upset stomach, elevated blood pressure, [and/or] chest pains" (p. 3).

The stress you experience can be a limiting factor, mental and physical, that doesn't allow you to express yourself among your peers. That expression can be attractive to other peers who want to get to know you. Stress can be an impediment to recovery success by impeding peer interactions, individual success, and personal expression.

Peer Experience: Stress

Stressors that come from interactions with peers demonstrate how important they are to healing after head injury. The important thing is to decide how best you can deal with stress. Personal stress reactions can signal a need for support from others who notice, or which interferes with a comfort level because it is conflicting with personal expression.

Stress can signal different stressors from the traumatic experience. It is feedback on how it is personally affecting you. Look at the symptoms that you are experiencing. Then ask what is personally calming to you or if you have any stress relief patterns.

The stress you feel indicates the importance you may be mentally putting on the event or trauma reacting to the situation. Find a way to support yourself through the stress of experiencing a traumatic situation.

THERAPY V. REHABILITATION

Therapy and rehabilitation are two sides of the same coin. While therapy may consist of performing exercises to get the body into shape, rehabilitation seeks to restore abilities held by the individual prior to the head injury. The mind-set of rehabilitation is finding success by returning to a previous version of yourself, getting back into shape, finding things that will restore you to how you were before the head injury occurred.

Therapy, on the other hand, is about strengthening who you are becoming, about adjusting to the individual circumstances that you are experiencing now. It is beginning to realize that while it would be great to re-enter the situation you had before the head injury, it may be good for you to decide that you are, in essence, starting anew.

Things become overwhelming when you begin to look at the rehabilitation processes required

---

117 Stupart (2018). Stress Affects College Students' Performance. Retrieved on: 5-26-2018. Retrieved from: https://owlcation.com/academia/College-Life-The-Effects-of-Stress-on-Academic-Perform...

to get back to your "old" life. The life that didn't include having a head injury experience. To enter a mind-set of rehabilitation and find the desire to get your abilities back to the functioning abilities you had before the head injury is to accept some presuppositions that your life is not supposed to be as it is now. Discovering what your life is now, as you are living it, is the optimal way to deal with challenges and situations that may feel like they are out of control. Therapy is done to prepare for the challenges ahead. Rehabilitation is done to get back to a situation that existed before the head injury.

Trying to attain that person you were before can add a huge mental strain. Enjoy the journey of your life. The experiences we go through are what mold our bodies and minds.

Consider looking at relationships as both rehabilitation and therapy. You will be working with who you are and participating in becoming a better, more prepared version of yourself. The relationships will help you become better while working with who you need to be. Become the person the relationships you participate in can make you be.

Peer Experience: Therapy v. Rehabilitation

The experience of a peer relationship brings therapeutic readiness and rehabilitative healing. By being involved in a relationship, your brain is healing. Entering a relationship provides therapeutic skills that enable finding success and a feeling of comfort and healing.

Relationships will nurture the individual struggling to heal from the trauma it has sustained. The longer you are in a relationship, the more self-healing skills you will acquire. The relationships you acquire will enable you to gain new skills (therapy), heal, and restore a state of health (rehabilitation). Peer relationships—they are therapy and rehabilitation. And they're waiting for you.

TRAUMA AND RELATIONSHIPS

The trauma experienced reflects the time the trauma happened and what parts of the individual psyche were affected. Feelings of violation and vulnerability reflect changes in worldview and feelings that show trauma's effects. According to the International Society for Traumatic Stress Studies (ISTSS),[118] "Trauma survivors may feel intense shame, unlovable, or bad in some way, or guilty about what happened to them or about something that they did or feel that they should have done in the traumatic situation" (p. 2).

The experiences of trauma can affect attachments in early life.[119] "…disrupted…attachments

---

118 International Society for Traumatic Stress Studies (n.d.). Trauma and Relationships. Retrieved 5-26-2018. Retrieved from: https: ISTSS_Main/media/Documents/ISTSS_TraumaAndRelationships_FNL.pdf

119 International Society for Traumatic Stress Studies (n.d.). Trauma and Relationships. Retrieved 5-26-2018. Retrieved from: https: ISTSS_Main/media/Documents/ISTSS_TraumaAndRelationships_FNL.pdf.

affect the person's ability to feel calm and to expect caring, responsive, comforting connections in adult life. Memories of betrayal, loss, shame, secrecy, violation, and threats to bodily integrity may surface or become part of later relationships" (p. 3).

Difficulties with trauma and relationships are multifaceted. Yet according to ISTSS,[120] "Treatment is available to respond to these difficult experiences, minimize isolation, and restore a sense of hope. It can be helpful to discuss traumatic experiences, feelings of grief, and relationship difficulties with a professional who is familiar with the complex effects of trauma" (p. 4).

The difficulties of engaging in relationships show the dichotomous association between trauma survivors and their need for a relationship to start healing. It is so easy to see the effects of trauma on an individual, yet it is so difficult to find the healing relationships that can encourage recovery.

Peer Experience: Trauma and Relationships

Overcoming the symptoms of trauma can be an overwhelming and frustrating process. The realizations of what trauma has changed will be daunting. So many different ways of feeling are possible, so many new ways of disrupted attachments manifesting into unsatisfying and unfulfilling relationships. Treatment with a professional can restore a sense of hope, of direction, and ultimately lay the pathway of finding satisfying relationships by overcoming manifestations of trauma.

Trauma is one of the most confusing and disarming senses of losing relationship opportunities. But if it is approached proactively with acceptance, the effects of trauma on relationships can be mitigated.

ULTIMATE SUCCESS FORMULA

Progress and the feedback which allows success to be understood make a powerful approach to healing from trauma. According to Shemp,[121]

1. "Know your outcome. Be specific in WHAT you want!
2. Know your WHY. When you know your why, the how's will work itself out. (sic)
3. Take massive action.
4. Know what you're getting. You need to assess your progress. If you want to lose weight and body fat, you need to measure before you start, each Monday and at the end.

---

120 International Society for Traumatic Stress Studies (n.d.). Trauma and Relationships. Retrieved 5-26-2018. Retrieved from: https: ISTSS_Main/media/Documents/ISTSS_TraumaAndRelationships_FNL.pdf.

121 Shamp (2016). Tony Robbins 5 Step Ultimate Success Formula (for any goal). Retrieved on: 5-29-2018. Retrieved from: http://brienshamp.com/2016/12/01/tony-robbins-5-step-formula/.

5. Change your approach. Based on your assessment of your progress, you may need to work on some strategies or beliefs. If you have hit a plateau or find yourself spiraling downhill, this is the time to ask for help. Spiraling often happen (sic) because we missed our opportunity to assess and missed the plateau that happened before the spiral" (p. 2).

The Ultimate Success is easiest expressed by asking yourself: What do you **WANT** to achieve?

What do you want?
Action you need to take
Notice if the plan is working
Tailor your approach to achieve what you want

By using the Ultimate Success Formula, you enable the process of finding success! Taking action and then reviewing feedback to see if any alterations need to be made can enhance skills for peer relationships!

Peer Experience: Ultimate Success Formula

By engaging in the Ultimate Success Formula, you bring a tool that will change difficulty with peer relationships to surprising sources of feedback! What do you WANT to improve on or experience? The Ultimate Success Formula can take you there!

UTILIZING PSYCHOANALYTICAL PRINCIPLES

Understanding relationships by principles that explain certain behaviors, according to Gans,[122] is obtained from analyzing "The Structural Model of Personality…personality is composed of three elements. These three elements of personality—known as the id, ego, and superego—work together to create complex human behaviors" (p. 1).

These elements that drive behaviors take precedence in explaining relationship success. According to Gans,[123] "The id is driven by the pleasure principle, which strives for immediate gratification…" (p. 1).

Relationships are not easy. Many of them require repeated tries and struggle. The longitudinal approach can be advantageous to relationships. But when the id is involved, participation in relationships will revolve around gratification, and that can distract you from being involved and

---

122 Gans (2017). What Are The Id, Ego, and Superego?. Retrieved on 5-30-2018. Retrieved from: https://www.verywellmind.com/the-id-ego-and-superego-2795951.

123 Gans (2017). What Are The Id, Ego, and Superego?. Retrieved on 5-30-2018. Retrieved from: https://www.verywellmind.com/the-id-ego-and-superego-2795951.

cognitively engaged in a relationship.

Another aspect of the psychoanalytic elements is the ego. According to McLeod,[124] "The ego develops to mediate between the unrealistic id and the external world" (p. 3). The id is reality. It deals with constraints and opportunities of what is possible.

The superego is another psychoanalytic element.[125] "The superego incorporates the values and morals of society which are learned from…others" (p. 4).

The superego can determine how peer relationships impact motivation and expressions. The ego demonstrates the constraints of society. What society expects or allows determines and predicts societal treatment of others and relationships.

The ego stands between the pulls of the id and the superego. The ego knows what reality allows between the two—instant gratification for the id, or relenting to find oneself constantly trying for approval from one's peers. Utilizing psychoanalytic principles is a way to truly interpret how relationship priorities can be met.

Peer Experience: Utilizing Psychoanalytic Principles

The aspects of a peer experience are often expressed in terms of the id, the ego, and the superego. The id is constantly wanting to express itself, to gratify itself. Rather than asking about another's day and expressing interest, the id wants to talk about what it is experiencing. Competing aspects of the common reality of self and others is revealed within the struggle for self-expression. The ego feels the pull of the id and the superego, and struggles to achieve a quantity of satisfying each of the aspects.

But regardless of how each element is satisfied, the pull of the three elements will always have a motivating appeal. How we spend the time we have demonstrates the current mindset that is being operated from. Healing from trauma, the aspect of the superego may play an overriding factor in your recovery.

Vicarious Experiences

The learning examples from our peers can serve as indicators of personal development. Looking at how a friend may be positively received and asking, "Why can't I do that?" is a definite indicator that your development is ready to improve by watching what your peers are doing; you are ready to copy what actions they are performing to find the results they are receiving. According to Peer Relations and Learning-Peer Relationships, Learning Motivation and Relationships, Classroom

---

124 McLeod (2016). Id, Ego, and Superego. Retrieved on: 6-1-2018. Retrieved from: https://www.simplypsychology.org/psyche.html.
125 McLeod (2016). Id, Ego, and Superego. Retrieved on: 6-1-2018. Retrieved from: https://www.simplypsychology.org/psyche.html.

Dynamics,[126] "…a developmental theory [exists] describing the changes in interpersonal needs as an individual matures" (p. 1). The predisposition to rely on peer models will reflect on the position that recovery allows us to see and attend to the abilities that we want to have. Learning and peer relationships are essentially linked. According to Peer Relations and Learning-Peer Relationships, Learning Motivation and Relationships, Classroom Dynamics,[127] "The peer group is an essential element in motivation and learning" (p. 2).

The most encouraging and motivating learning can come from the foundation of peer experience.[128] "[Learners] are not isolated in the pursuit of knowledge. They are social beings who need to interact and establish social contacts. Social learning is as much a part of any classroom curriculum as the printed guidelines. At a minimum, the influence of peers and…relationships with them can be understood as a function of…age, motivation, learning, and…opportunities" (p. 3).

Peer Experience: Vicarious Experiences

The attention each individual exhibits to their peer group will signal their readiness as a vicarious learner. As important as learning vicariously can be in peer learning, the most essential realization that needs to come about is an individual's ability to easily transition into peer roles that will reflect their development as a person with respect to their trauma.

The most important realization is the effect of trauma on the individual that also affects the motivational aspects of how peers may be viewed or allowed to be teachers of the peer skills that will increase recovery ability and trauma resilience.

VISUALIZATION

Complications interfere with recovery and rehabilitations from head injury. Disabilities may impede successful demonstrations of key recovery concepts. Most importantly, the experience of learning from the demonstration of these skills is taken from you when the environment is not ready for you to demonstrate your skills. There needs to be another way that allows successful use and experience of peer skills. The skill of visualization allows you to, according to Adams,[129] "…practice your golf swing, work out your muscles, prepare to climb Mount Kilimanjaro, hone your chess skills, practice for tomorrow's surgery, and you can even prepare for your best life!" (p. 1).

---

126 Peer Relationships and Learning—Peer Relationships, Learning Motivation and Relationships, Classroom Dynamics. (n.d.). Retrieved on: 6-1-2018. Retrieved from: http://education.stateuniversity.com/pages/2315/Peer-Relations-Learning.html

127 Peer Relationships and Learning—Peer Relationships, Learning Motivation and Relationships, Classroom Dynamics. (n.d.). Retrieved on: 6-1-2018. Retrieved from: http://education.stateuniversity.com/pages/2315/Peer-Relations-Learning.html.

128 Peer Relationships and Learning—Peer Relationships, Learning Motivation and Relationships, Classroom Dynamics. (n.d.). Retrieved on: 6-1-2018. Retrieved from: http://education.stateuniversity.com/pages/2315/Peer-Relations-Learning.html.

129 Adams (2009). Seeing Is Believing: The Power of Visualization. Retrieved on 5-30-2018. Retrieved from: https://www.psychology today.com/us/blog/flourish/200912/seeing-is-believing-the-power-…

Peer relationships carry a lot of variables. Perceptions of others about your personal abilities can never be accurately interpreted. Regardless, according to Adams,[130] "Mental practice can get you closer…where you want to be in life, and it can prepare you for success!" (p. 1).

Are visualizations truly effective? How can mentally visualizing something be as effective as really doing something? Yet, doing visualizations can increase the predisposition of a person to perform the skills visualized. Visualizations can come closer to reality than what might be expected. According to Adams,[131] "Research has revealed that mental practice is almost as effective as true physical practice and that doing both is more effective than either alone" (p. 1).

Research reports,[132] "…Thoughts produce the same mental instructions as actions. Mental imagery impacts many cognitive processes of the brain: motor control, attention, perception, planning, and memory. So the brain is getting trained for actual performance during visualization… Mental practices enhance motivation, increase confidence and self-efficacy, improve motor performance, prime your brain for success…all relevant to achieving your best life!" (p. 2).

Visualization can be the ultimate rehabilitation exercise. The final step is learning how to make your visualization the most effective it can be! According to Adams,[133] "Hold a mental 'picture' as if it were occurring to you right at that moment. Imagine the scene in as much detail as possible. Engage as many of the five senses as you can in your visualization. Who are you with? Which emotions are you feeling right now? What are you wearing? Is there a smell in the air? What do you hear? What is your environment? Sit with a straight spine when you do this. Practice at night or in the morning… Eliminate any doubts… Repeat this practice often. Combine with meditation or an affirmation (e.g., 'I am courageous; I am strong')" (p. 2).

Peer Experience: Visualization

Visualizations can reproduce and enhance the peer experience. By adding them to your learning, you enable your brain to be introduced to peer situations it may be yearning to learn. Enhance your peer experience with visualizations!

---

130 Adams (2009). Seeing Is Believing: The Power of Visualization. Retrieved on 5-30-2018. Retrieved from: https://www.psycholo-gytoday.com/us/blog/flourish/200912/seeing-is-believing-the-power-…

131 Adams (2009). Seeing Is Believing: The Power of Visualization, Retrieved on 5-30-2018. Retrieved from: https://www.psycholo-gytoday.com/us/blog/flourish/200912/seeing-is-believing-the-power-…

132 Adams (2009). Seeing Is Believing: The Power of Visualization. Retrieved on 5-30-2018. Retrieved from: https://www.psycholo-gytoday.com/us/blog/flourish/200912/seeing-is-believing-the-power-…

133 Adams (2009). Seeing Is Believing: The Power of Visualization. Retrieved on 5-30-2018. Retrieved from: https://www.psycholo-gytoday.com/us/blog/flourish/200912/seeing-is-believing-the-power-…

Water Intake for the Brain

Water actually provides the cognitive abilities for the success of recovery. It provides clarity and abilities that are needed with peer skills and for recovery and rehabilitation from head injury. According to Hearn & Hearn,[134] "Drinking water and brain function are integrally linked. Lack of water…can cause numerous symptoms including problems with focus, memory, brain fatigue, and brain fog, as well as headaches, sleep issues, anger, depression, and many more" (p. 1).

The symptoms of not getting enough water are pretty severe, but even more important is choosing to drink water for the energy the brain needs. According to Hearn & Hearn,[135] "…Brain cells need two times more energy than other cells in the body. Water provides this energy more effectively than any other substance" (p. 1). Using the power of water,[136] "you will be able to think faster, be more focused, and experience greater clarity and creativity" (p. 2).

Hydration has become so casual that it is reduced to when opportunity strikes. Yet it is more important than that. Grabbing a drink of water may be reduced to the idea of when you see the next water fountain, you can take the opportunity to drink. According to Hearn and Hearn,[137] "The reason why it is so important to drink plenty of water throughout the day for optimal brain function is because your brain does not have any way to store water" (p. 2). Schedule water breaks in your day to influence your brain performance. Because your peer relationships and recovery deserve it.

Peer Experience: Water Intake for the Brain

The next time you are enjoying a great time with your peers, pay attention to the amount of water you have had that day. When your responses are right on cue, when your thoughts are clear, and you are expressing yourself well, your brain has found the way to its own power probably by your choice to hydrate. Choose water when needing a boost to your mental activity!

---

134 Hearn & Hearn (2018). Water and Brain Function How to Improve Memory and Focus. Retrieved on: 5-30-2018. Retrieved from: https://www.waterbenefitshealth.com/water-and-brain.html.

135 Hearn & Hearn (2018). Water and Brain Function How to Improve Memory and Focus. Retrieved on: 5-30-2018. Retrieved from: https://www.waterbenefitshealth.com/water-and-brain.html.

136 Hearn & Hearn (2018). Water and Brain Function How to Improve Memory and Focus. Retrieved on: 5-30-2018. Retrieved from: https://www.waterbenefitshealth.com/water-and-brain.html.

137 Hearn & Hearn (2018). Water and Brain Function How to Improve Memory and Focus. Retrieved on: 5-30-2018. Retrieved from: https://www.waterbenefitshealth.com/water-and-brain.html.

WELLNESS

Wellness is represented by six areas for those trying to be well. The categories involve, according to the National Wellness Institute,[138] "emotional, occupational, physical, social, intellectual, [and] spiritual" (p. 1) areas of wellness. According to the National Wellness Institute,[139] "Wellness is defined by being a conscious, self-directed, and evolving process of achieving full potential… Wellness is multidimensional and holistic, encompassing lifestyle, mental and spiritual well-being, and the environment… Wellness is positive and affirming" (p. 2).

Utilizing wellness and its benefits allows awareness of[140] "[the] interconnectedness of each dimension…contribute to healthy living…" (p. 2). All aspects of wellness incorporate the idea of interconnection and being able to direct oneself to positive achievement. There is an amount of confidence that happens when living your life to be well. An individual who gives their recovery the best chance at wellness **POISES** themselves for greatness.

Their wellness gives them confidence and assuredness that they will be able to complete whatever they need to do.

POISES is:

Physical—Are you actively using your body and brain?

Occupational—Do you find some way of looking at yourself as skilled and contributing?

Intellectual—Do you have an emphasis on learning?

Social—Whom do you communicate with? Are you spending time with people who appreciate you?

Educational—Do you learn things? Not, do you learn things easily, just "are you learning?"

Spiritual—Connecting with sources that nourish your existence.

The concept of wellness revolves around a philosophy of self-direction enabling an interplay of different opportunities and attention, and how, according to the National Wellness Institute,[141] "… benefits of regular physical activity, healthy eating habits, strength and vitality as well as personal responsibility, self-care and when to seek medical attention" (p. 2). The aspects of wellness actually are beneficial to the individual by drawing attention to the aspects of a healthy life—participation

---

138 National Wellness Institute (n.d.). The Six Dimensions of Wellness. Retrieved on: 5-30-2018. Retrieved from: https://www.nationalwellness.org/general/custom.asp?page=Six_Dimensions.

139 National Wellness Institute (n.d.). The Six Dimensions of Wellness. Retrieved on: 5-30-2018. Retrieved from: https://www.nationalwellness.org/general/custom.asp?page=Six_Dimensions.

140 National Wellness Institute (n.d.). The Six Dimensions of Wellness. Retrieved on: 5-30-2018. Retrieved from: https://www.nationalwellness.org/general/custom.asp?page=Six_Dimensions.

141 National Wellness Institute (n.d.). The Six Dimensions of Wellness. Retrieved on: 5-30-2018. Retrieved from: https://www.nationalwellness.org/general/custom.asp?page=Six_Dimensions,

in a lifestyle that is balanced with wellness and that opens up recovery opportunities to those who are recovering from head injury.

Peer Experience: Wellness

The interconnection of aspects of wellness can influence recovery and rehabilitation. By attending to aspects of wellness and health that is contained within the categories of occupational, physical, social, intellectual, spiritual, and emotional well-being, the direction and attention actually take a wider perspective than just a simple aspect of doing therapy. The individual who practices wellness POISES well among those in recovery and rehabilitation.

Xenophobia

Xenophobia is limiting to recovery and causes people recovering from head injury to miss the healing interactions that come from strangers. If a person smiles and says hi to you but you choose to ignore them because they are not your friend, this may signal a definite leaning toward xenophobia. This missed interaction may also give you a chance to see where you are in your understanding the trauma that resides in you. A chance at healing is what every conversation holds. Talking to others can bring the affiliation that can heal, but if trauma is resounding strongly in ourselves, xenophobia will be the result. The definition of xenophobia is, according to Merriam-Webster,[142] "fear and hatred of strangers or of anything that is strange or foreign" (p. 1).

The ability to talk with strangers and make them your friends may not come easily to others. Many trauma survivors may even dislike the idea of befriending someone. Social support is proving to be so valuable, however, that the xenophobia must be overcome. Social support, according to Dougher, is[143] "…useful in helping individuals cope with stress" (p. 1).

Find the aspect of yourself that is fully alive and supported because of overcoming xenophobia. Choose to feel supported by communicating with others. Overcome the trauma from the head injury by reinforcing peer relationships.

---

142 Merriam-Webster (2018). Definition of Xenophobia. Retrieved on: 5-30-2018. Retrieved from: https://www.merriam-webster. com/dictionary/xenophobia.

143 Dougher (1985). Social support as a mediator of stress: Theoretical and empirical issues. Retrieved on: 5-30-2018. Retrieved from: https://www.sciencedirect.com/science/article/pii/027273588590039X.

> **Peer Experience: Xenophobia**
>
> **Many people are strange and foreign, until you get to know them. And then they become familiar and domestic. It is all a question of how you want to communicate with them to find support for yourself. Find who you can be without the trauma that is affecting you. Choose to supply the conversation that will heal you.**

X-RAY OF RECOVERY

To fully participate in a recovery, critical examination of the aspects of a successful recovery must be completed. A series of literature that emphasizes consistent applications of coping skills and adaptive mechanisms will allow recovery success.

The X-ray of recovery reveals that successful recovery from head injury requires:

1. First, supplying coma communication information from new research and using Maslow's Hierarchy to supply rehabilitation and recovery information for the body and brain's needs to understand what is fulfilling and practicing the habits that encourage self-sustenance.
2. Next, an emphasis on healing trauma with a relationship perspective to bring the healing of attachments.
3. Closing the opportunities of recovery, a book emphasizing the longitudinal changes in perspective to partially extend the view of a complete head injury recovery.
4. Finally, a book addressing trauma and finding a way to express it to reintegrate damaged hemispheres and be the concluding book to a head injury recovery.

1. *HEADS UP: From Coma to Completion*

   Many recoveries can start from an individual in a coma. Using breakthrough approaches toward understanding comas, *HEADS UP* uses adaptive approaches to influence learning essential skills, fulfilling the skills needed to add a feeling of recovery completion as your potential is discovered.

2. *ABCs of Head Injury: Peer-Oriented Skills for Recovery from Brain Injury*

   An intense analysis of healing factors and adaptive philosophies of trauma healing relationships. Understanding adaptive recovery approaches and bringing what the brain needs from the perspective of rehabilitation that can allow a better approach to recovery.

3. *Discovering Yourself: FLIGHT PLANS*

   A longitudinal approach to influencing recovery with different perspectives can encourage lasting approaches. Changing how recovery is viewed can encourage the person we discover within to use the most effective recovery approaches.

4. *Creative Healing: Healing Trauma with Creativity and Integration*

   Expressing trauma and reintegrating damaged hemispheres means healing trauma and expressing it to mold part of yourself. Powerful methods of healing happen when finding ways of producing with trauma.

YERKES-DODSON

The Yerkes-Dodson law is not just a small factor of performance; it is the function. According to Cherry,[144] "Yerkes-Dodson law suggests that elevated arousal [stress] levels can improve performance up to a certain point" (p. 1).

Performance is improved when you feel a touch of nerves that activate the brain's potential. According to Cherry,[145] "There is a relationship between performance and arousal. Increased arousal can help improve performance, but only to a certain point…" (p. 1). Approaching a relationship where you may be trying to speak to an individual you feel attracted to will actually enhance your performance, yet when you're feeling a crushing amount of stress that is activating your trauma and making communication impossible, you are not accessing the performance-enhancing potential of Yerkes-Dodson. You're just dealing with trauma and its deleterious effects.

By accessing the potential of Yerkes-Dodson, you can access the best of the brain's relationship

---

144 Cherry (2020). Yerkes-Dodson Law and Performance. Retrieved on 6-1-2018. Retrieved from: https://www.verywellmind.com/what-is-the-yerkes-dodsen-law-2796027.

145 Cherry (2020). Yerkes-Dodson Law and Performance. Retrieved on 6-1-2018. Retrieved from: https://www.verywellmind.com/what-is-the-yerkes-dodsen-law-2796027.

potential. But using Yerkes-Dodson does take self-monitoring and the ability to adjust the trauma with an application of slower breathing. Keep the stress and arousal within a "sweet spot" where you can still operate with the anxiety but which engages and awakens your brain to its best performance.

> **Peer Experience: Yerkes-Dodson Performance**
>
> **Being able to monitor personal experience and making use of deep breathing can help one deal with moderate trauma. The stress effect that comes from trauma is a different aspect than the nervousness that comes about from the Yerkes-Dodson performance. But, by self-monitoring and trauma control with a deep breathing pattern, the Yerkes-Dodson Law can be realized and your performance can be increased. Staying in the "sweet spot" of your brain will energize its performance because of positive stress to awaken it to its possibilities and find its top performance.**

YOGA

Yoga is a graceful, poised repetition of focused breathing that relies on concentration and balance to connect with the body and heal trauma. According to van der Kolk,[146] "Yoga can be a powerful element in healing trauma" (p. 2). Yoga contributes to community and support, and it is also an exercise that helps calm trauma survivors.[147] "When people are traumatized, they become afraid of their physical sensations, their breathing becomes shallow, and they become uptight and frightened about what they're feeling inside. When you slow down your breathing with yoga, you can increase your heart rate variability, and that decreases stress. Yoga opens you up to feeling every aspect of your body's sensations. It's a gentle, safe way for people to befriend their bodies, where the trauma of the past is stored" (p. 2).

Yoga incorporates the community of a group practice.[148] "…It's interesting that it's so much more satisfying to do yoga in a group than by yourself. There's a likelihood that doing yoga in groups may activate the mirror neuron system of the brain, which is a system damaged by trauma, so practicing yoga and meditation in groups might give people a deeper sense of belonging" (p. 3).

Resolving trauma shows a very specific treatment plan. According to van der Kolk,[149] "…Trauma is really a somatic issue. It's in your body and because of that yoga has great relevance, because it

146 van der Kolk (n.d.). Befriending Your Body: How Yoga Helps Heal Trauma. Retrieved on: 6-1-2018. Retrieved from: https: // kripalu.org/resources/befriending-your-body-how yoga helps-heal-trauma.

147 van der Kolk (n.d.). Befriending Your Body: How Yoga Helps Heal Trauma. Retrieved on: 6-1-2018. Retrieved from: https: // kripalu.org/resources/befriending-your-body-how yoga helps-heal-trauma.

148 van der Kolk (n.d.). Befriending Your Body: How Yoga Helps Heal Trauma. Retrieved on: 6-1-2018. Retrieved from: https: // kripalu.org/resources/befriending-your-body-how yoga helps-heal-trauma.

149 van der Kolk (n.d.). Befriending Your Body: How Yoga Helps Heal Trauma. Retrieved on: 6-1-2018. Retrieved from: https: // kripalu.org/resources/befriending-your-body-how yoga helps-heal-trauma.

goes directly to sensing and befriending the body. …The most important part is starting to regain ownership of your body and be comfortable in your own skin" (p. 2). Yoga as a treatment for trauma shows a great deal of promise.[150] "…Yoga is equally as beneficial—or more beneficial—than the best possible medications in alleviating traumatic stress symptoms" (p. 2).

Peer Experience: Yoga

Dealing with trauma, yoga may be the best way to try to soothe your nerves. It is some of the best medicine to engage in and find a practice that calms trauma. Find a chance that allows you to find focus at re-experiencing your body. Finding belonging and finding a deeper purpose are just some of the effects of yoga. It's time to lose your yourself in the possibilities of discovering yoga and how it can be the best treatment for your trauma.

FINDING THE ZONE

Peak performance is what keeps each human striving to discover who they are. The "zone" allows humanity to, according to McNamara,[151] "…capture the essence of the human spirit and showcase human potential" (p. 1). Finding the zone is essential for humans to achieve their best. It can be found in five easy steps. But how does anyone **CATCH** the zone?

To find the zone and unearth human potential, according to McNamara,[152] you need:

Confidence—Confidence is "the cornerstone of success in all domains of life, and developing it is much like nurturing a garden'" (p. 1). Nurturing the confident ability frees the inner passion which connects the brain with doing its best.

A moment—The moment we take allows ascertaining the situation which may need a response. According to McNamara,[153] "Take a moment before going to bed to think about a question or important situation to dream about. This can lead to dreams that unmask hidden obstacles and clarify issues" (p. 2).

Total synchronicity—The zone combines thoughts and actions and actions to work and solve problems.[154] "The Zone is 'a mental state in which your thoughts and actions are occurring in complete synchronicity.' Entering it enables you to perform at your highest level" (p. 2).

---

150 van der Kolk (n.d.). Befriending Your Body: How Yoga Helps Heal Trauma. Retrieved on: 6-1-2018. Retrieved from: https: // kripalu.org/resources/befriending-your-body-how yoga helps-heal-trauma.

151 McNamara (2008). 5 Things We Learned From Finding Your Zone: Ten Core Lessons for Achieving Peak Performance in Sports and Life. Retrieved on 5-30-2018. Retrieved from: http://articles.chicagotribune.com/2008-08/10/features/0808060330_sports-and-life-zone…

152 McNamara (2008). 5 Things We Learned From Finding Your Zone: Ten Core Lessons for Achieving Peak Performance in Sports and Life. Retrieved on 5-30-2018. Retrieved from: http://articles.chicagotribune.com/2008-08/10/features/0808060330_sports-and-life-zone…

153 McNamara (2008). 5 Things We Learned From Finding Your Zone: Ten Core Lessons for Achieving Peak Performance in Sports and Life. Retrieved on 5-30-2018. Retrieved from: http://articles.chicagotribune.com/2008-08/10/features/0808060330_sports-and-life-zone…

154 McNamara (2008). 5 Things We Learned From Finding Your Zone: Ten Core Lessons for Achieving Peak Performance in Sports and Life. Retrieved on 5-30-2018. Retrieved from: http://articles.chicagotribune.com/2008-08/10/features/0808060330_sports-and-life-zone…

Concentration—By focusing in on performing a skill, the variability of success is reduced to its highest quality. According to McNamara,[155] "The best way to practice a skill is to limit the focus to the task at hand" (p. 2).

Here and now—The most amazing part of the zone is believing you are prepared and your readiness has allowed you to come to this point and succeed.[156] "…You have prepared yourself… to perform" (p. 2). The zone is a special place that culminates with your experiences that have prepared you to be your best.

Peer Experience: Finding the Zone

The zone is an amazing place in which to operate and a liberating place for individual abilities. It allows the human spirit to be seen and the best of relationships to be achieved. When finding the preparation and confidence, the human spirit becomes a showcase of potential. Relationships form, people admire your abilities, and you become the legend that your life has always had the potential to be.

The zone is available to everyone, yet few people have the opportunity to CATCH it. By returning to the zone and increasing your potential, you bring a new standard of performing to who you are.

ZENITH OF RECOVERY

The height of your recovery is extending to heal your injuries. Every achievement of recovering personal skills will influence brain injury and enable a survivor to get that much closer to their potential. Recovery skills build off each other, pushing the essence of the human spirit and demonstrating and eclipsing human potential. The recovery potential that you dream about and hope to one day achieve is here. You are doing it. Combining communication skills with peers, influencing attachments, and healing trauma allow the best of belonging and self. There is no other place to go.

You have completed the second book of the four-book series. Are you ready to go on, or is this your zenith of recovery? What you choose is perfect for you.

---

155 McNamara (2008). 5 Things We Learned From Finding Your Zone: Ten Core Lessons for Achieving Peak Performance in Sports and Life. Retrieved on 5-30-2018. Retrieved from: http://articles.chicagotribune.com/2008-08/10/features/0808060330_sports-and-life-zone...
156 McNamara (2008). 5 Things We Learned From Finding Your Zone: Ten Core Lessons for Achieving Peak Performance in Sports and Life. Retrieved on 5-30-2018. Retrieved from: http://articles.chicagotribune.com/2008-08/10/features/0808060330_sports-and-life-zone...

Peer Experience: Zenith of Recovery

The choices you make from here on out will continue your success. The legacy you continue to build with your advancing progress is what makes the zenith of recovery; you are exactly where you are supposed to be. The choice to push recovery further is what makes you able to stand where you are right now. It's not the climb to the zenith of recovery that makes the recovery from a head injury so impressive: it's the fact that you've made it as far as you have and that you choose to look where you've been and now are choosing to be satisfied with where you are. Congratulations. You have made it as far as you have needed to.

LOVE—SEPARATE ENTITIES: A NEW *CREATURE*

The difference between singles who are dating and couples in love is a reliance and connection with each other. It changes from two individuals to one identity: a different **CREATURE** altogether. Love and relationships can be a hard recipe to follow, depending on what part of the brain has been injured and the corresponding changes in abilities. The abilities that we each are challenged to replicate result in a difference in relationship abilities. Changed abilities means a relationship can be hard to establish and fulfill. But establishing a new **CREATURE** that incorporates the skills of each of the relationship partners means the growth of a loving relationship. Starting with the "couple bubble," we begin to see the identity of a loving partnership and new forms of reliance and commitment. Love begins to be a new **CREATURE:**

Couple bubble—The relationship that you have with another starts with the couple bubble that you form between yourselves. A couple bubble is what allows feelings of love, emotional investment, and happiness. According to Pappenheim,[157] "…You have a powerful platform for…trust and…intimacy and happiness in your love relationship" (p. 1). The struggle within the couple bubble is each partner viewing themselves as individuals. According to Pappenheim,[158] couples struggle with their views of their dependence. They start by "…seeing themselves as individuals first, and as a couple very much second" (p. 2). The couple bubble[159] is emphasized by "positive dependency…couples were able to admit their needs and empathize with each other…fostering …a loving, safe environment in which each supports and nurtures…" (p. 3). The couple bubble rests on the pact of[160] "we come first" (p. 4).

Relating to your partner—Your choice to demonstrate knowledge of what your partner wants

---

157 Pappenheim (n.d). How To Fix A Relationship With A "Couple Bubble." Retrieved on 6-6-18. Retrieved from: https://livebold-andbloom.com/11/relationships/how-to-fix-a-relationship.

158 Pappenheim (n.d). How To Fix A Relationship With A "Couple Bubble." Retrieved on 6-6-18. Retrieved from: https://livebold-andbloom.com/11/relationships/how-to-fix-a-relationship.

159 Pappenheim (n.d). How To Fix A Relationship With A "Couple Bubble." Retrieved on 6-6-18. Retrieved from: https://livebold-andbloom.com/11/relationships/how-to-fix-a-relationship.

160 Pappenheim (n.d). How To Fix A Relationship With A "Couple Bubble." Retrieved on 6-6-18. Retrieved from: https://livebold-andbloom.com/11/relationships/how-to-fix-a-relationship.

or needs, according to Young,[161] "…self-management, knowledge of your partner…" (p. 2), is very important. Observing, appreciating, relating, and having empathy for your partner as well as having the ability to deliver consistent applications of caring and self-control will encourage a relationship to grow and change how it needs to.

Expertise on pleasing and soothing a partner—Pleasing and soothing your relationship partner can be very special. According to Healthy Relationship Advice,[162] "Sex in relationships can truly be divine" (p. 1). The intimacy that solidifies the relationship is truly special. This concept is about cultivating an expertise in partner enjoyment and arousal—in other words, knowing the pleasure points that your partner desires.

Avoid war and make love—The art of relationships is about knowing a partner's time to be loved and to receive their loving when they decide to give it. Disagreements or fighting will not be a time to express loving for your partner or talk about the minutia of a relationship that you may need to resolve. What has to occur in a relationship, according to Francis,[163] is that "every emotion has an appropriate time and healthy modes of expression" (p. 1). Pick your time and place, but when you are fighting, it is not a good time for loving actions.

Third party avoidance—Partners should work to maintain the exclusivity in a relationship. This means preventing third parties from becoming more important to you than your partner. According to Towner,[164] third parties do have status in a relationship. "…The importance that other people play in a romantic love relationship…. couple relationships that include other people are necessary for its survival, but they can also pose threats to the love relationship itself… anywhere from annoying to toxic…" (p. 1). Being a couple that is strengthened by third party avoidance and even more reliant upon themselves is important. Positive dependency is enhanced as functioning with another couple can increase a couple's dependence on each other.

Using rituals in relationships—Relationships can benefit from the use of rituals. Discussions of rituals, according to the Gottman Institute,[165] reveal "'rituals of connection'…an important tool for successful relationships. A ritual of connection is a way of regularly turning towards your partner that can be counted on" (p. 1). Rituals of connection bring a consistent and dependable way to bring feelings of love and allow using a type of schedule of reinforcement.

Rekindling love with just one glance—Eye contact is one of the most important ways to see love's

---

161 Young (2017). What's the Secret to a [sic] Being a Happy Couple? Retrieved on: 6-6-2018.. Retrieved from: https://www.in-dewpendent.co.uklife-style/love-sex/happy-relationship-love-skills-communic...

162 Healthy Relationship Advice (n.d.). Healthy Relationship Advice. Retrieved on: 6-6-2018. Retrieved from: https://www.healthy-relationship-advice.com/sex-in-relationships.html.

163 Francis (2017). How Honoring Negative Emotions Can Heal. Retrieved on: 6-6-2018. Retrieved from: https://thebody isnota-napology.com/magazine/the-importance-of-anger/.

164 Towner (2017). 52 Ways: What Motivates Others Who Threaten a Relationship? Retrieved on 6-6-2018. Retrieved from: www.psychologytoday.com/us/blog/life-refracted/201711/52-ways-what-motivates-o...

165 The Gottman Institute (n.d.). 5 Rituals to Reconnect In Your Relationship. Retrieved on 6-6-2018. Retrieved from: https://www.gottman.com/blog/5-rituals-reconnect-relationship/.

possibilities. According to Rizzo,[166] "…The eyes are not just windows to the soul, but also neuron pathways that can form love connections… Eye contact is a way of feeling connected, and feeling that [another person] is interested in you has a huge effect of feeling love for that person" (p. 2).

Emphasis on the fulfillment and satisfaction of relationships—Finding fulfillment in a loving relationship is not just a simple matter of "being born" with the skill. According to Psychology Today,[167] "Love is one of the most profound emotions known to human beings. There are many kinds of love, but most people seek its expression in a romantic relationship with a compatible partner. For some, romantic relationships are the most meaningful element of life, providing a source of great fulfillment. The ability to have a healthy, loving relationship is not innate. A great deal of evidence suggests that the ability to form a stable relationship [requires us] to work consciously to master the skills necessary to make them flourish" (p. 1). The most important, fulfilling love relationship depends on what is made into the relationship for each of us.

Peer Experience: CREATURE

The experience of bringing two separate entities together in a platonic or sexual relationship depends on the CREATURE acronym. The couple bubble is essential for all relationships—it's the trust, investment, and belief you have in yourselves that make the relationship. Relating to your relationship partner involves accepting who they are. Expertise with being pleasant or being able to soothe your partner deals with the comfort you feel between yourselves and being aware of stress levels. Avoiding war and finding love and happiness are essential to find moments where you don't struggle but have happy times between yourselves. Third party avoidance allows you to both enjoy each other for your own gifts. Using rituals could be as simple as going out to celebrate an achievement at a favorite place or watching a favorite TV program together. Emphasis on the goodness of a relationship is as simple as maintaining the relationship by continuing to keep ideas of your next meeting so you can help sustain the relationship. Find the creature you can with your relationship proficiency!

SEXUAL EXPRESSION AND RELATIONSHIPS

A romantic relationship can be one of the biggest stressors in a person's life, be that as positive (as a motivator) or negative (as a demotivator). It can provide a great source of joy in someone's life as well. Regardless of whether you are currently in a relationship, sexuality is something that each of us carries with us in our personality. Considering these factors, it is crucial that we examine the

---

166 Rizzo (n.d.). Can Eye Contact Make You Fall in Love? Retrieved on 6-6-2018. Retrieved from: https://www.theguardian.com/intimacy-secrets-for-all/2017/jun/01/can-eye-contact-make-y...

167 Relationships: All About Relationships (n.d.). Retrieved on 6-6-2018. Retrieved from: https://www.psychologytoday.com/us/basics/relationships.

value of sexuality and sexual expression in your recovery.

The important discovery about sexual expression and disability is stated clearly by Disabled World:[168] "Sexuality is an integral part of the personality of everyone, man, woman, and child: it is a basic need and aspect of being human that cannot be separated from other aspects of life" (p. 1). Sexuality is important to people's expression and individuality.

Disability is a tricky subject. Factors such as misunderstanding and ignorance intrude into conversation about disability and sexuality, and many people with disabilities may be turned away from even thinking about themselves as sexual. Society demonstrates an intolerance of differences and places enormous positive value and emphasis on having a perfect body. To be imperfect is to be asexual and anonymous or overlooked in the sexual spectrum of life. Yet, by adopting the saying **I DARED TO BELIEVE** there is a relationship for me, sexuality can be considered.

Invest in yourself—A commitment to and belief in yourself is essential to your expression of yourself as a disabled person. According to Disabled World,[169] "…A disability does not alter the right of an individual to express his or her sexuality" (p. 3).

Develop good sexual communication skills—Good sexual communication can correct, according to Disabled World,[170] "difficulties in social and personal development" (p. 2).

Actively engage—People with disabilities benefit from keeping actively involved in interests and activities which can serve as things to talk about to others or topics of interest.

Risk social rejection—Trying to make new friends and relationships by introducing yourself to someone new is a needed aspect of overcoming the constraints of having a disability.

Entertain your sexual side—This can be done by various means: reading erotica, fantasizing, and reading information. According to Disabled World,[171] "…People with disabilities often find reading erotic literature can help spark the imagination as well as the libido" (p. 2).

Decide to seek out advice, counselling or psychotherapy—Talking about issues can be helpful to overcoming[172] "…sexual issues that may be associated with their particular disability."

Try not to overcompensate—Self-doubts and insecurities may come to a head during relationship attempts. These stressful times can exacerbate different compensatory behaviors.

Open sharing of information—According to Disabled World,[173] many myths say [people with disabilities] "don't need sexuality education" (p. 2).

---

168 Disabled World (n.d.) Disability Sexuality: Sex and the Disabled Information. Retrieved on: 6-11-2018. Retrieved from: https://www.disabledworld.com/disability/sexuality/.
169 Disabled World (n.d.) Disability Sexuality: Sex and the Disabled Information. Retrieved on: 6-11-2018. Retrieved from: https://www.disabledworld.com/disability/sexuality/.
170 Disabled World (n.d.) Disability Sexuality: Sex and the Disabled Information. Retrieved on: 6-11-2018. Retrieved from: https://www.disabledworld.com/disability/sexuality/.
171 Disabled World (n.d.) Disability Sexuality: Sex and the Disabled Information. Retrieved on: 6-11-2018. Retrieved from: https://www.disabledworld.com/disability/sexuality/.
172 Disabled World (n.d.) Disability Sexuality: Sex and the Disabled Information. Retrieved on: 6-11-2018. Retrieved from: https://www.disabledworld.com/disability/sexuality/.
173 Disabled World (n.d.) Disability Sexuality: Sex and the Disabled Information. Retrieved on: 6-11-2018. Retrieved from: https://www.disabledworld.com/disability/sexuality/.

Behave lovingly—Having a disability actually minimalizes an individual who is in a relationship, yet it is so important to not let the disability affect the love you express.

Emotionally satisfied—Trying not to be emotionally needy, according to Disability World,[174] "people with….disability…have...fulfilling…lives…" (p. 2).

Listen actively—Relationships need interested partners, both in communication and responsiveness. By listening actively, you allow yourself to engage with your partner.

Interesting and informed—By keeping informed about topics that could serve as interesting conversation, you allow yourself to know your partner better and for them to know you.

Educate yourself—Many people with disabilities may need to inform themselves. According to Disabled World,[175] "According to one survey, up to 50% of adults with disabilities are not in any sexual relationship at all. Online disabled dating sites…specifically aimed at people with disabilities have been founded to fill this void" (p. 3).

Very positive outlook—Relationships for people with disabilities benefit from a positive outlook that will guide them and provide positive opportunities.

Enjoying others—The reality of relationships is that whatever your personal situation, it is increased by the ability to enjoy others, and your happiness contributes to the relationship!!

Peer Relationships: I DARED TO BELIEVE

Having a disability is definitely a challenge to a relationship. But by maintaining the skills included in I DARED TO BELIEVE, relationships are enhanced and encouraged! In fact, by practicing these skills, I am enjoying the results of continuing a relationship with much success!

WHAT ARE YOUR LETTERS?

What are the letters that have connected you to having an idea of a relationship? What do you see as working well for you, and helping you heal the trauma within? What makes a healing relationship a possibility?

---

174 Disabled World (n.d.) Disability Sexuality: Sex and the Disabled Information. Retrieved on: 6-11-2018. Retrieved from: https://www.disabledworld.com/disability/sexuality/.

175 Disabled World (n.d.) Disability Sexuality: Sex and the Disabled Information. Retrieved on: 6-11-2018. Retrieved from: https://www.disabledworld.com/disability/sexuality/.

Index